Phytotherapy in The Management of Diabetes and Hypertension

(Volume 4)

Edited by

Mohamed Eddouks

Faculty of Sciences and Techniques Errachidia
Moulay Ismail University of Meknes
Errachidia
Morocco

Phytotherapy in the Management of Diabetes and Hypertension

Volume # 4

Editor: Mohamed Eddouks

ISSN (Online): 2452-3232

ISSN (Print): 2452-3224

ISBN (Online): 978-981-14-8051-5

ISBN (Print): 978-981-14-8049-2

ISBN (Paperback): 978-981-14-8050-8

need for a court order if at any point you breach any terms of this License Agreement. In no event will any delay or failure by Bentham Science Publishers in enforcing your compliance with this License Agreement constitute a waiver of any of its rights.

3. You acknowledge that you have read this License Agreement, and agree to be bound by its terms and conditions. To the extent that any other terms and conditions presented on any website of Bentham Science Publishers conflict with, or are inconsistent with, the terms and conditions set out in this License Agreement, you acknowledge that the terms and conditions set out in this License Agreement shall prevail.

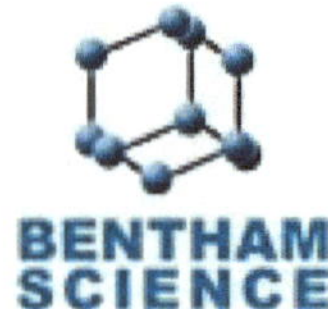

CONTENTS

PREFACE

In order to provide an up-to-date overview of the phytotherapy of diabetes and hypertension, this fourth volume has been prepared as part of the ebook series "Phytotherapy in the Management of Diabetes and Hypertension". The present volume includes different aspects of the pathophysiology of diabetes and hypertension. This book adds important information related to the evaluation of the efficacy and safety of medicinal plants and their derivatives on diabetes and hypertension. The present volume includes 6 complementary chapters presenting an updates on clinical study reports of phytotherapy in the management of type 2 diabetes mellitus; curcumin: a drug of choice for the treatment of diabetes and hypertension; olive leaf, a traditional phytomedicine for diabetes and hypertension; medicinal plants from genus *Costus* in management of diabetes; antidiabetic and antihypertensive potential of *passiflora* SPP (passion fruit) - an updated review and monograph on *Anvillea radiata* Cross. & Durieu. This volume will be useful to the students, teachers, researchers, scientists, clinicians and even the common people.

ACKNOWLEDGMENTS AND GRANTS

The Editor would like to thank all the authors and the reviewers for their contribution to this volume. This work was supported by the Ministry of National Education, Vocational Training, Higher Education and the Scientific Research (Morocco) and the National Center for Scientific and Technical Research (CNRST) (Morocco) under grant N° PPR/2015/35.

Mohamed Eddouks
Faculty of Sciences and Techniques Errachidia
Moulay Ismail University of Meknes
Errachidia
Morocco

List of Contributors

Adeeb Shehzad	Department of Pharmacy, Institute for Research and Medical Consultations, Imam Abdulrahman Bin Faisal University, Dammam, Saudi Arabia
Anil Bhanudas Gaikwad	Department of Pharmacy, Birla Institute of Technology and Science, Pilani, Pilani Campus Pilani- 333031, Rajasthan, India
Ankit P. Laddha	Shobhaben Pratapbhai Patel School of Pharmacy & Technology Management, SVKM's NMIMS, V.L. Mehta Road, Vile Parle (West), Mumbai-400056, India
Bency Baby T.	Department of Pharmacogosy, Al Shifa College of Pharmacy, Perintalmanna, Kerala - 679 325, India
Ebtesam A. Al-Suhaimi	Department of Biology, College of Science, Imam Abdulrahman Bin Faisal University, Dammam, Saudi Arabia
Flavio Francini	CENEXA; UNLP-CONICET CCT La Plata-FCM; CEAS-CICPBA, La Plata, Argentina
Guillermo R. Schinella	Cátedra de Farmacología Básica, Facultad de Ciencias Médicas, UNLP, CICPBA, La Plata, Argentina
Isabel Andújar	Departament de Farmacologia, Universitat de València, Spain
José Luis Ríos	Departament de Farmacologia, Universitat de València, Spain
Kaveri M. Adki	Shobhaben Pratapbhai Patel School of Pharmacy & Technology Management, SVKM's NMIMS, V.L. Mehta Road, Vile Parle (West), Mumbai-400056, India
Luisa González-Arbeláez	Centro de Investigaciones Cardiovasculares, CCT UNLP-CONICET, La Plata, Argentina
Mahfuza Afroz Soma	Department of Pharmacy, State University of Bangladesh, 77 Satmasjid Road, Dhaka 1205, Bangladesh
Manisha J. Oza	Shobhaben Pratapbhai Patel School of Pharmacy & Technology Management, SVKM's NMIMS, V.L. Mehta Road, Vile Parle (West), Mumbai-400056, India
Md. Moklesur Rahman Sarker	Department of Pharmacy, State University of Bangladesh, 77 Satmasjid Road, Dhaka 1205, Bangladesh
Meneerah A. Aljafary	Department of Biology, College of Science, Imam Abdulrahman Bin Faisal University, Dammam, Saudi Arabia
Mohamed Eddouks	Faculty of Sciences and Techniques Errachidia, Moulay Ismail University of Meknes, BP 509, Boutalamine, 52000, Errachidia, Morocco
Mourad Akdad	Faculty of Sciences and Techniques Errachidia, Moulay Ismail University of Meknes, BP 509, Boutalamine, 52000. Errachidia, Morocco
Raheem Shahzad	Department of Biology, College of Science, Imam Abdulrahman Bin Faisal University, Dammam, Saudi Arabia
T.N.K. Suriyaprakash	Department of Pharmaceutics, Al Shifa College of Pharmacy, Perintalmanna, Kerala - 679 325, India
Yogesh A. Kulkarni	Shobhaben Pratapbhai Patel School of Pharmacy & Technology Management, SVKM's NMIMS, V.L. Mehta Road, Vile Parle (West), Mumbai-400056, India

CHAPTER 1

Updates on Clinical Study Reports of Phytotherapy in the Management of Type 2 Diabetes Mellitus

Md. Moklesur Rahman Sarker[1,2,*] and **Mahfuza Afroz Soma**[1]

[1] *Department of Pharmacy, State University of Bangladesh, 77 Satmasjid Road, Dhaka 1205, Bangladesh*

[2] *Health Med Science Research Limited, 3/1 Block F, Lalmatia, Dhaka 1207, Bangladesh*

Abstract: Type 2 diabetes mellitus (T2DM) is a metabolic disorder caused by the insufficient production of insulin and/or the development of resistance to insulin. The long-term management of T2DM with conventional oral hypoglycaemic drugs is a challenge as these drugs may worsen certain underlying comorbidities and complications, such as chronic kidney and cardiovascular diseases. Besides, because of the development of resistance to those drugs, it is difficult to control hyperglycemia for long term treatment of type 2 diabetes mellitus patients. This drawback of conventional medicines necessitates phytotherapy, herbal medicines, functional foods, nutraceuticals, and other forms of alternative medicines or the invention of new medicines for the effective and long term treatment of type 2 diabetes mellitus avoiding the major adverse-effects or minimising them. Plant-derived bioactive compounds are a great resource for the discovery of new medicines. Besides, phytomedicines in the forms of extracts, isolated compounds, combined herbal preparations or other forms can be used for the prevention and treatment of type 2 diabetes mellitus. This chapter contains updated panorama based on the evidences from clinical study reports on different forms of phytotherapy, including plant extracts, its fractions, isolated bioactive compounds, functional foods, nutraceuticals, herbal medicines formulations and other forms of plant-derived phytotherapy reported for the treatment of type 2 diabetes mellitus. The findings from clinical study reports were discussed with proper citations as well as presented in summarized form in a table. A total of 52 different types and forms of prospective phytomedicines, bioactive compounds, or formulation or extracts or fractions or decoctions or functional foods formulations having clinical study reports associated with type 2 diabetes mellitus were presented in this chapter. The molecular mechanisms involved along with the primary and secondary outcomes with phytotherapy on type 2 diabetes patients were also presented. Multiple clinical studies demonstrated very prospective and potential antidiabetic activities of Berberine, Bitter gourd, Cinnamon, Curcumin, Dia-Best™, Fenugreek, Gegen Qinlian decoction, GlucoSupreme herbal, *Gymnema sylvestre*, Magnesium, *Nigella sativa*, Resveratrol,

---

* **Corresponding author Prof. Md. Moklesur Rahman Sarker:** Professor and Head of Academic & Research, Department of Pharmacy, State University of Bangladesh, 77 Satmasjid Road, Dhaka 1205, Bangladesh; Chief Researcher, Health Med Science Research Limited, 3/1 Block F, Lalmatia, Dhaka 1207, Bangladesh; Tel: +8801776758882; E-mail: moklesur2002@yahoo.com & dr.moklesur2014@gmail.com

Mohamed Eddouks (Ed.)

Tibetan medicine herb combination, TCM multiple herbal combination, Xiaoke pill, and vitamin C. Hence, at least, these phytoremedies are recommended for the management of type 2 diabetes mellitus which may have additional benefits in diabetes management compared to conventional Allopathic medicines considering the long-term safety and effectivity of the products. The updated clinical study reports on phytotherapy presented in this chapter will be helpful for the medical, biological and pharmaceutical researchers and complementary and alternative medicine users to use these plants extracts, its fractions, isolated biomolecules, herbal preparations, functional foods, nutraceuticals and other forms of phytomedicines for the prevention and treatment of diseases as well as for the discovery of modern medicines.

Keywords: Bioactive Compounds, Clinical studies, Complementay and alternative medicine, Herbal medicine, Phytomedicine, Phytotherapy, Type 2 diabetes mellitus.

INTRODUCTION

Diabetes mellitus is a group of metabolic disorders characterized by high blood glucose levels. Diabetes mellitus is caused by insufficient or absence of insulin production or impairment of insulin action or both, which results with the disturbances of the metabolism of carbohydrate, protein, and fat [1]. Diabetes is classified into the following categories:

1. Type 1 diabetes mellitus (also called insulin-dependent diabetes): This occurs due to the destruction of pancreatic β-cells by autoimmunity, which leads to the complete deficiency of insulin production.
2. Type 2 diabetes mellitus (also known as non-insulin dependent diabetes): This occurs because of the progressive loss of insulin production or secretion from pancreatic β-cells or the development of resistance to insulin or because of both reasons.
3. Gestational diabetes mellitus (GDM): GDM occurs because of the hormonal and metabolic changes of pregnant women, and is diagnosed in the second or third trimester of pregnancy.
4. Specific types of diabetes: Diabetes may also be developed due to other specific reasons, such as i) monogenic diabetes syndromes: neonatal diabetes and maturity-onset diabetes of the young, ii) diseases of the exocrine pancreas: cystic fibrosis and pancreatitis, iii) drug- or chemical-induced diabetes: glucocorticoid use in the treatment of HIV/AIDS or after organ transplantation [1, 2].

Diabetes can be diagnosed by measuring fasting plasma glucose (FPG) or post-prandial plasma glucose two hours after meal (2-h PG) level or glycated hemoglobin A_1C (HbA1c) criteria [2]. People with FPG $\geq$ 7.0 mmol/L, 2-h PG $\geq$

11.1 mmol/L, HbA1c $\geq$ 6.5%, or random blood glucose $\geq$ 11.1 mmol/L in the presence of signs and symptoms are diagnosed to have diabetes [1, 3].

The prevalence and incidence of diabetes is increasing all over the world irrespective of lower-income, middle-income and developed countries. According to WHO 2018 report, the number of diabetic patients has increased from 108 million in 1980 to 422 million in 2014 [4].The global prevalence of diabetes in adults over 18 years of age has increased from 4.7% in 1980 to 8.5% in 2014 [4]. According to the report of the International Diabetic Association in 2017, approximately 425 million adults (20-79 years) were reported to live with diabetes, which is estimated to be raised to 629 million by 2045 [5]. It was found that the highest number of diabetes patients was between the age of 40-59 years, and 50% (212 million) of the people with diabetes were undiagnosed [5]. In the year 2017, more than 1.1065 million children were found to live with type 1 diabetes mellitus, and 352 million people were at risk of developing type 2 diabetes mellitus around the globe [5]. It is also noteworthy to mention here that IDF reported 79% of adults with diabetes were living in low- and middle-income countries [5].

According to WHO report 2018, an estimated 1.6 million deaths were directly caused by diabetes in 2016 and diabetes was found to be the seventh leading cause of death [4]. Diabetes is a major cause of cardiovascular diseases such as, heart attacks and stroke, kidney failure, blindness [4]. Chronic diabetes state causes severe consequences with heart attacks, stroke, blindness (due to damage to the small blood vessels in the retina), damage nerves, causes the risk of obesity, erectile dysfunction, foot ulcers, infections, kidney failure, cancer and ultimately death of the patients [1, 4, 6, 7].

The current treatment options for diabetes mellitus are oral hypoglycemic drugs and injectables, mainly insulin. Oral antihyperglycemic drugs are classified as follows:

1. Biguanides (Example: metformin): American Diabetic Association recommends metformin as the first line oral drug for the treatment of type 2 diabetes mellitus. Metformin reduces hepatic gluconeogenesis and lipogenesis, decreases intestinal absorption of glucose, and improves insulin sensitivity by increasing peripheral glucose uptake and utilization [8 - 10].
2. Sulfonylureas (Examples: Glimepiride, glipizide, gliclazide): Sulfonylureas are known as insulin secretagogues because of this class of antidiabetic drugs induces the secretion of insulin from pancreatic beta-cells. American Sulfonylureas are recommended as a classic second-line therapy for the treatment of type 2 diabetes mellitus. Sulfonylureas increases insulin secretion

regulated by ATP-sensitive potassium channels located in the membrane of beta cells of the pancreas [9, 11].

3. Meglitinides (Examples: Repaglinide, nateglinide): Meglitinides are another type of oral insulin secretagogues. Meglitinides increase insulin secretion by a mechanism similar to that of sulfonylureas, but with more rapid absorption and more rapid stimulus to insulin secretion, with a shorter half-life. The insulin secretion is regulated by ATP-sensitive potassium channels located in the membrane of beta cells of the pancreas but having a different subunit of the binding site at the membrane of beta cells [9, 11, 12].

4. α-Glucosidase inhibitors (Examples: Acarbose, miglitol, voglibose): α-glucosidase inhibitors competitively inhibit membrane-bound intestinal alpha-glucoside enzymes responsible for the digestion of dietary starch in the intestine. This causes delayed carbohydrate absorption and digestion, inhibits the reabsorption of polysaccharides as well as the metabolism of sucrose to glucose and fructose and results in a reduction in postprandial hyperglycaemia [9, 11].

5. Thiazolidinediones (rosiglitazone, pioglitazone): Thiazolidinediones bind to peroxisome proliferator-activated receptor gamma (PPAR-γ), which is predominantly found in the central nervous system, adipose tissue and pancreatic beta-cells, to increase the sensitivity of insulin. This class of drugs thus increases peripheral uptake of glucose and decrease hepatic glucose production [9, 11].

6. Dipeptidyl peptidase - 4 (DPP-4) inhibitors (sitagliptin, saxagliptin, vildagliptin, linagliptin, alogliptin): The incretin hormones - glucagon like peptide-1 (GLP-1) and gastric inhibitory polypeptide (GIP), secreted by intestinal L cells, increase insulin secretion, inhibits the secretion of glucagon, decrease gastric emptying, and nourish the health of beta-cells of the pancreas. DPP-4 rapidly inactivates those incretin hormones. DPP-4 inhibitors inhibit DPP-4 enzymes, and thus facilitate to perform the activity of those two incretin hormones for a long time. By doing so, the DPP-4 inhibitors reduce glucose levels in plasma and improve islet function and health in type 2 diabetes mellitus patients [9, 11].

7. Sodium glucose co-transporter2 (SGLT2) inhibitors (dapagliflozin and canagliflozin): SGLT2 inhibitors block sodium-glucose cotransporter 2 in proximal tubules of renal glomeruli which causes inhibition of 90% glucose reabsorption. This results an increase in glycosuria and diuresis in people with type 2 diabetes mellitus, which in turn reduces the plasma glucose levels, weight, and blood pressure [9, 11].

The long-term management of type 2 diabetes mellitus (T2DM) with conventional oral hypoglycaemic drugs is a challenge as these drugs may worsen certain underlying comorbidities and complications, such as chronic kidney and cardiovascular diseases. Besides, because of the development of resistance to those drugs, it is difficult to control hyperglycemia for long term treatment of diabetes patients. This drawback of conventional medicines necessitates phytotherapy, herbal medicines, functional foods, nutraceuticals and other forms of alternative medicines or the invention of new drug molecules for the effective and long term treatment of T2DM avoiding the major adverse-effects and minimising the minor side-effects. Many experimental evidences proved the pharmacological and therapeutic potentiality and scientific basis of medicinal plants, phytocompounds, herbal preparations, functional foods and other forms of phytomedicines for use in the prevention and treatment of different diseases including diabetes [13 - 16], cancer [17, 18], immunity [19 - 23], obesity and hyperlipidemia [15, 24], oxidation, inflammation [25] and infections [26]. Plant-derived bioactive compounds are a great resource for the discovery of new medicines. Besides, the phytomedicines in the forms of extracts, isolated compounds or other forms can be used for the prevention and treatment of T2DM. This chapter contains the updated evidences from clinical study reports on different forms of phytotherapy, including plant extracts, its fractions, isolated bioactive compounds, functional foods, nutraceuticals, herbal medicines formulations and other forms of plant-derived phytoremedies reported to be beneficial in the treatment of T2DM. The functional mechanism of different forms of phytomedicines exhibited in clinical studies on type 2 diabetes patients is presented in Fig. **(1)**.

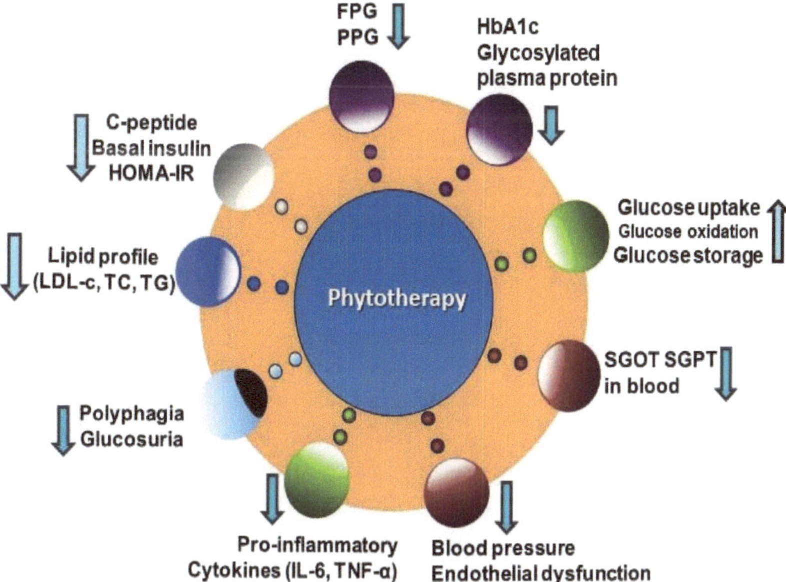

Fig. (1). Functional mechanism of phytotherapy in clinical studies on Type 2 diabetes mellitus patients.

The updated clinical study reports on phytotherapy presented in this chapter will be helpful for the medical, biological and pharmaceutical researchers and complementary and alternative medicine practitioners and users to consider the use the potential plants extracts, its fractions, isolated biomolecules, herbal preparations, functional foods, nutraceuticals and other forms of phytomedicines for the prevention and treatment of diseases as well as for the discovery of modern medicines.

METHODOLOGY TO SEARCH ARTICLES

In order to collect relevant information on clinical trials or clinical study reports on Phytotherapy, articles were searched systematically using the PubMed (https://www.ncbi.nlm.nih.gov/pubmed/) search engine for accessing the MEDLINE database, Science Direct, Wiley Online Library, Clinicaltrials.org, Google scholar and Google using the following terms: "Phytotherapy for diabetes research" and "Clinical trials of phytotherapy for diabetes". All the relevant articles, published in the English language between 1970 and August 2019, were collected for extensive review to write this book chapter.

Clinical Study Reports of Phytoremedies in Diabetes Mellitus Patients

The clinical study reports of different phytomedicines for the treatment of diabetes mellitus have been presented in Table **1** in addition to the details study report of each phytomedicine described below:

Aloe vera

Aloe vera, belongs to the Liliaceae family, is a traditional remedy for diabetes in the Arabian Peninsula [27]. Aloe gel is made from the inner portion of the *Aloe vera* leaf. The leaf contains glucomannan fiber, which may have prospective hypoglycemic effects [28]. In 1996, the same researcher group reported improved fasting blood glucose levels by conducting two nonrandomized clinical trials (n=76 and n=40) administering aloe gel for 6 weeks [29, 30]. Another trial using half a teaspoonful aloe gel daily was conducted among five type 2 diabetic patients for 4-14 weeks and showed a reduction in fasting blood glucose and HbA1c level [31]. A randomized, double-blind, placebo-controlled clinical trial asserted a significant decrease in fasting blood glucose, HbA1c, total cholesterol, and LDL levels two months after administering two 300 mg capsules aloe gel along with two 5 mg glyburide tablets and two 500 mg metformin tablets daily. This trial was conducted to assess the potency of these drug combinations among 30 type 2 diabetic patients aged from 40 to 60 years who were hyperlipidemic and did not take anti-hyperlipidemic agents [32].

Alpha-lipoic Acid

α-lipoic acid is a naturally occurring fatty acid and also a potent antioxidant. A multiple-dosage controlled trial was reported to have significant glucose uptake and insulin sensitivity without changing fasting blood glucose level. This trial randomly selected seventy-four patients with type 2 diabetes and among them, 19 were administered placebo whereas the rest were divided into three test groups with active treatment of α-lipoic acid in various doses daily, *i.e*, 600 mg once (n=19), twice (n=18), or thrice (n=18) for 4 weeks [33]. Konrad *et al.* performed a noncontrolled trial and compared serum lactate and pyruvate levels of diabetic patients with those of lean (n=10) and obese (n=10) healthy subjects after glucose loading. This trial showed the efficacy of α-lipoic acid in impeding hyperglycemia-induced rise of serum lactate and pyruvate levels [34].

Artocarpus heterophyllus and *Asteracanthus longifolia*

In 1991, Fernando MR *et al.* carried out a short-term non-randomized, open-label study on 20 maturity-onset diabetic patients and 20 healthy human subjects to assess the efficacy of hot-water extracts of *Artocarpus heterophyllus* leaves and *Asteracanthus longifolia* whole plant material. Both the extracts showed positive effects on glucose tolerance in the healthy subjects and the diabetic patients when 200 mL decoction, prepared from 200g fresh leaves, was administered as a single dose prior to performing GTT [35].

Bellpepper *(Capsicum annuum* var. Grossum) Juice

Nagasukeerthi *et al.* conducted a randomized controlled study on fifty T2DM patients who were divided into either study group (receiving 100 mL of bell pepper juice (twice/day) combined with an integrated approach of yoga therapy (IAYT)) or control group (receiving only IAYT) for 4-consecutive days. The study reported a significant reduction in post prandial blood glucose, systolic blood pressure, pulse pressure, rate pressure product and double product in the study group compared with control group [36].

Berberine from *Berberis aristata*

Several plants, for example, *Berberis* genus and *Coptis chinensis* yielded an isoquinoline alkaloid, which is called Berberine. Yin *et al.* carried out two trials to evaluate the efficacy of berberine (500 mg, three times a day) isolated from *Berberis aristata* on T2DM patients for three months. The first trial was conducted on newly diagnosed T2DM patients administering berberine or metformin. The trial exhibited a similar outcome of berberine and metformin monotherapy in reducing HbA1c, FPG, postprandial glucose, basal insulin and postprandial insulin. The second trial reported significant improvement in different parameters, like-HbA1c, FPG, PBG, basal insulin, homeostasis model assessment of insulin resistance (HOMA-IR), fasting C-peptide and postprandial C-peptide after administering berberine as adjuvant therapy in poorly controlled T2DM patients [37]. Zhang *et al.* also conducted a randomized, double-blind, placebo-controlled trial for 3 months using berberine (1000 mg daily). A significant decrease in HbA1c, FPG and PBG was observed among berberine group compared with the placebo group. Moreover, HbA1c reduction in test group was comparable to that of the present oral hypoglycemic drugs [38]. In 2010, another trial displayed improved insulin sensitivity using 1000 mg of berberine daily, which indicated berberine as a potent antidiabetic agent compared with metformin or rosiglitazone. This trial also showed the effectiveness of this alkaloid in maintaining a glycemic profile in patients suffering from hepatitis, whereas some current antidiabetic agents, like metformin and rosiglitazone have shown hepatic side effects [39]. Another study performed by Gu *et al.* (2010), also verified the effects of berberine as antihyperglycemic and antihyperlipidemic agent administering 1000 mg/day of berberine for three-months [40]. A trial was carried out in patients with 5.6-7.5 baseline HbA1c level co-morbid with non-alcoholic fatty liver disease using treatments include life style intervention (LSI) alone or combined with berberine or pioglitazone for 4 months. Significant reduction was found in HbA1c along with other glycemic parameters in combination therapy rather than LSI only, which were similar to that of pioglitazone [41]. However, the potential effects of berberine (900 mg/d) on glycemic, lipidemic, and anthropometric parameters as well as the inflammatory parameters including CPR, LPS, and TNF-α were ascertained after a two month trial on T2DM patients [42]. In 2018, Lazavi F *et al.* performed a randomized clinical trial feeding with 200 ml barberry juice (BJ) daily for eight weeks. Total Cholesterol and triglyceride level were significantly reduced in BJ group [43].

Berberol

Berberol is a nutraceutical mixture made from *Berberis aristata* extract (588 mg, standardized based on 85% berberine), and *Silybum marianum* extract (105 mg, standardized based on 60% flavonolignans) [44]. In 2012, Di Pierro *et al.* performed a clinical trial on T2DM patients with trivial glycemic control using berberol two times a day for three months. HbA1c, basal insulin and HOMA-IR were significantly decreased. The outcomes of this trial indicated that berberol could be a potential supplement to increase insulin sensitivity [45]. Di Pierro *et al.* (2013) conducted another trial administering berberine (1000 mg/d) or berberol (two times a day) in two separate groups of T2DM patients for 4 months. Both formulations significantly reduced HbA1c and FPG; however, berberol was more potent in reducing HbA1c level than berberine. SGOT and SGPT were also reduced, which is similar to the previous trial [46]. In 2015, another study was carried out to assess the effectiveness of berberol in 45 hypercholesterolemic T2DM patients with statin intolerance for 12 months. All the patients were divided into three groups: control group (n=15) who were not taking hypolipidemic drugs due to a recent diagnosis of hypercholesterolemia and statin intolerance; 15 were diagnosed with hypercholesterolemia and treated with ezetimibe (10 mg/day) due to statin intolerance diagnosed in the previous year; 15 were being treated with low doses of statins due to a diagnosed intolerance to high-dosage statins. Significant improvement in HbA1c and FPG, as well as lipid profile, were found in all groups of patients without any serious side effects [47].

Bitter Gourd *(Momordica charantia)*

Active components of *Momordica charantia* (balsam pear/karolla/bitter gourd/bitter melon) are charantin, vicine, and polypeptide-p (unidentified insulin-like protein resembles bovine insulin) [48]. Welihinda *et al.* reported strong beneficial effects of *M. charantia* fruit juice (100 ml, 30 min before the oral glucose load) on blood glucose by performing a short-term controlled metabolic trial on 18 type 2 diabetic patients [49]. In another trial, nine patients were administered with subcutaneous vegetable insulin extract (purified protein extract of fruits and tissue cultures of *M. charantia*), which was shown to have a consistent hypoglycaemic effect with no hypersensitivity reaction to this extract. The onset of action of this plant insulin was within 30-60 min with the peak effect six hours after the administration [50]. A 4-week, multicenter, randomized, double-blind, active-control trial was carried out among 120 patients with type 2 diabetes. The patients were divided into 4 groups administering bitter melon 500 mg/day, 1000 mg/day, and 2000 mg/day or metformin 1000 mg/day. The findings of the trial indicated that the dosage 2000 mg/day of bitter melon possessed modest hypoglycemic effect as well as significantly decreased fructosamine levels [51]. Another systematic review has been performed using bitter gourd preparations by Peter *et al.*, which also confirmed that these preparations have beneficial effects in lowering elevated fasting plasma glucose in prediabetes [52].

Carnitine

Carnitine or its derivative acetyl-L-carnitine was given to type 2 diabetic patients to evaluate its efficacy in improving blood glucose levels. Three small controlled short-term metabolic trials were found that revealed the positive effects of intravenous carnitine administration (n=18, n=15, and n=9) in enhancing insulin sensitivity as well as glucose uptake and storage [53 - 55].

Caucasian Whortleberry (*Vaccinium arctostaphylos* L.)

Mirfeizi *et al.* performed a randomized triple-blinded clinical trial on 105 T2DM patients using 1000 mg/day cinnamon (n=30), 1000 mg/day Caucasian whortleberry (n=30) and 1000 mg/day starch (placebo group, n=45) for 3 months. Both cinnamon and whortleberry significantly reduced FBG, 2-h PPG, insulin serum, HbA1c, and HOMA-IR levels in diabetic patients compared to the placebo group [56].

Celery *(Apium graveolens* L.*)*

In a randomized clinical trial, Yusni *et al.* (2018) found promising improvement in pre-prandial and post-prandial plasma glucose levels after treating 16 elderly pre-diabetic patients with celery leaf (capsules obtained from *A. graveolens* leaf extract at the dose of 250 mg, 3 times per day) for 12 days [57].

Chromium

Chromium (Cr_3) has potent hypoglycemic activity and its trivalent form is required to maintain glucose metabolism. A double-blind, placebo-controlled, crossover study was performed on 30 T2DM patients receiving either chromium picolinate or placebo for 2 months. This trial showed a significant decrease in triglyceride levels without any significant difference between the control and chromium-treated subjects in glucose control, high-density lipoprotein cholesterol levels, or low-density lipoprotein cholesterol levels [58]. In a double-blind, randomized clinical trial, chromium picolinate treated group showed a significant reduction in fasting and 2-h insulin levels after 2 and 4 months supplementation. The trial enrolled 180 type 2 diabetic patients and divided them into three groups administering either placebo, or 1.92 µmol (100 µg) Cr as chromium picolinate two times per day, or 9.6 µmol (500 µg) Cr two times per day [59]. 29 obese subjects who have family history of Type 2 diabetes were allocated randomly in two groups in a double-blind, randomized, placebo-controlled trial for 8 months. The subjects were treated with either 1,000 µg/day chromium picolinate (CrPic) or placebo. Chromium picolinate displayed significant improvement in insulin sensitivity [60]. Another double-blind, randomized, cross-over study enrolled seventy eight type 2 diabetic patients administering either Brewer's yeast (23.3 ug Cr/day), or $CrCl_3$ (200 ug Cr/day) sequentially with placebo in between, comprised of four stages, each lasting 8 weeks. Different blood glucose parameters like- fasting and 2 hour post glucose level, fructosamine as well as triglycerides levels were found to decrease significantly after supplementation with both the doses [61]. Another trial was conducted to evaluate the efficacy of yeast containing a high amount of chromium (160µg/d in 4 pellets) supplementation in elderly subjects (n=26) with stable impaired glucose tolerance.

However, there was no improvement in glucose tolerance or serum lipid levels [62]. Anderson *et al.* (1991) showed that supplemental chromium (chromium chloride; 200µg/d) caused significant improvements in glucose, insulin, and glucagon variables in subjects with marginally elevated blood glucose [63]. In 1992, Abraham *et al.* performed a trial on 25 patients with stable non-insuli--dependent diabetes mellitus administering daily with either 250 µg of chromium orally (chromium chloride) or a placebo for a period of 7 to 16 months. They revealed that there was no considerable change in fasting blood glucose level in diabetic or nondiabetic subjects after chromium supplementation for periods of up to 16 months [64]. However, Anderson *et al.* (2001) suggested the potential antioxidant effects of the individual and combined supplementation of Zn and Cr in 110 type 2 DM patients [65].

Cinnamon (*Cinnamomum zeylanicum*)

Cinnamon has been extensively studied for its therapeutic efficacy and safety in clinical trials. A meta-analysis of 10 randomized controlled trials which included 543 patients with type 2 diabetes mellitus and used cinnamon (*Cinnamomum zeylanicum*) doses starting from 120 mg to 6 g per day in different clinical studies for a period of four to eighteen weeks resulted with the reduction of fasting plasma glucose (-24.59 mg/dL), total cholesterol (–15.60 mg/dL), LDL-C (–9.42 mg/dL) and triglycerides (–29.59 mg/dL) levels, and increased the levels of HDL-C (1.66 mg/dL) in diabetes patients. But cinnamon could not significantly reduce the HbA1c levels (–0.16%) in diabetes patients [66]. In a 4 months double-blind randomized trial, 79 type 2 diabetes mellitus patients, taking oral antidiabetics or diet, were allocated to take either the cinnamon extract (3 g of cinnamon powder) or a placebo capsule (three times) daily. The findings of this trial showed that cinnamon extract significantly decreased the blood glucose level in cinnamon group (10·3%) comparing to placebo group (3·4%) without any adverse-effect [67].

Coccinia indica

The coccinia powder is obtained from crushed freeze-dried leaves of *Coccinia indica*. The powder was reported to have significant effects in improving blood glucose level among poorly controlled or untreated type 2 diabetic patients (*n*=32) after 6 weeks of administration, in a double-blind control trial, conducted in 1979 [68]. In another controlled clinical trial, pellets made from fresh dried leaves were used to compare its efficacy with a conventional hypoglycemic drug (chlopropamide) on 70 type 2 diabetic patients for 12 weeks. The findings showed that the herb ameliorated different blood glucose parameters similar to that of the drug [69]. Kamble SM *et al.* revealed that *C. indica* acts like insulin in an open-label trial following six weeks' use of dried extract of the herb orally in 30 diabetic patients at a dose of 500 mg/kg body weight [70].

Corn Bran (Zea Species)

Hanai *et al.* (1997) suggested that low dose supplementation with soluble corn bran hemicellulose (CBH) has potential effects in glycemic control. They carried out a long-term trial to observe the efficacy of soluble CBH (10g/day) on three groups: patients with impaired glucose tolerance (IGT) with (n=20) or without (n=8) obesity and healthy non-obese controls (n=10) for 6 months. CBH significantly reduced HbA1c in the obese patients, however, the fasting glucose level also reduced in all the groups, but not significantly [71].

Curcumin from *Curcuma longa* (Turmeric)

Curcumin is a polyphenol yielded from the rhizome of *Curcuma longa* L. (turmeric). In 2008, changes in HbA_1c and lipid profile were not significant in a randomized, placebo-controlled, parallel-group trial conducted among three groups of patients: curcumin 300 mg/d (23 patients) *vs.* atorvastatin 10 mg/d (23 patents) *vs.* placebo (21 patients) for 2 months [72]. The same dosage of curcumin was used in another trial for 3 months. HbA1c, triacylglycerol (TAG) and free fatty acid (FFA) level were significantly reduced in curcumin-treated group in comparison to the placebo group [73]. A double-blind randomized clinical trial allocated 70 patients with type-2 diabetes receiving either curcumin (80 mg nano-micelle formulation daily) or placebo for 3 months. Curcumin treated group was found to have a significant decrease in HbA1c, TAG, TC, and BMI [74].

Curcuminoids (Turmeric) Plus Piperine

In 2017, Panahi *et al.* conducted a 12-weeks double-blind, placebo-controlled study in which 118 patients with T2D were randomly divided to administer either curcuminoids (1000 mg/day plus piperine 10 mg/day) or placebo (plus standard of care) to evaluate the efficacy of supplementation with curcuminoids plus piperine in controlling serum lipids. Curcuminoids decreased serum levels of atherogenic lipid indices, including non-HDL-C and lipoprotein (a) (Lp(a)), which may lead to alleviating the risk of cardiovascular events in dyslipidemic T2DM patients [75].

Dia-Best™

Dia-Best™ is a commercially available polyherbal dietary supplement which contains a combination of Cinnamon bark (*Cinnamomum zeylanicum*), Fenugreek seed (*Trigonella foenum-graceum*), *Nigella sativa* seed, Oat, *Ganoderma lucidum*, and Bitter gourd powder. A single blind prospective intervention study was conducted by Sarker *et al.* (2019) on 30 uncontrolled type 2 diabetes mellitus patients receiving oral medications and/or insulin, age between 30-70 years old, with or without other complications, were orally administered with 1 sachet of Dia-Best powder (3g powder/sachet) in the morning 20 minutes before breakfast and at night 1 hour before sleep 60 days. After 2 months, the fasting blood glucose level was decreased from 11.63 mmoL/L to 8.92 mmoL/L (23.30%, p<0.001), HbA1c level from 8.9% to 7.2% (19.1%, p<0.001) as well. The glucose tolerance test showed significant reduction (29.70%, p<0.001) in post-prandial blood glucose levels (19.66 to 13.82 mmoL/L) 2-hours after meal. Total serum cholesterol (p<0.01), low density lipoprotein (LDL-c) (p<0.01), and triglyceride (TG) (p<0.001) levels were also significantly improved. No considerable adverse-effect was observed in any patient [76].

Fenugreek *(Trigonella foenum-graecum)*

There are several trials available for *Trigonella foenum-graecum* (fenugreek) in type 2 diabetes. In 1990, Sharma *et al.* performed a short-term randomized, cross over trial among 15 patients with non-insulin dependent diabetes (10 days). The patients were administered diets with or without 100 g of defatted fenugreek seed powder. Diet with fenugreek significantly reduced fasting blood glucose levels and showed improvement in glucose tolerance test as well as insulin responses. Another 20 days study displayed similar changes of higher magnitude in all the above parameters using fenugreek seeds in the diets of 5 diabetic patients [77]. The same research group conducted another randomized, controlled study in which type 1 diabetic patients were administered 100 g defatted fenugreek seed powder. The dosage was divided into two equal doses and served with diets during lunch and dinner. Fenugreek showed significant fall in fasting blood glucose and improvement in the glucose tolerance test [78]. Moreover, several short-term randomized crossover trials were carried out among 38 healthy subjects giving different preparations of fenugreek before oral GTT. The trials used whole raw seeds, extracted seed powder, gum isolate of seeds, and cooked whole seeds and the outcomes resulted in reduced postprandial glucose levels, but degummed seeds and cooked leaves did not show any improvement [79]. An open-label study indicated beneficial effects of fenugreek seed (15 g) in controlling blood glucose level on 21 T2DM patients for 6 months [80]. In 2008, Fu-rong *et al.* enrolled 69 patients with poor blood glucose levels taking oral sulfonylureas. The patients were randomly divided into two groups: the treated group (46 cases) having fenugreek (0.35 g/pill) and the control group (23 cases) having placebo three times daily (each time 6 pills) for 12 weeks. FBG, 2-h post-prandial blood glucose and HbA1c levels were significantly reduced in the fenugreek treated group as compared to those in the control group [81].

Ficus carica

Serraclara *et al.* (1998) investigated the efficacy of tea obtained from fig leaf (*Ficus carica*) in glycemic control in a crossover study. After 4 weeks, 10 type 1 diabetic patients were found to have reduced postprandial glucose and insulin requirements without reducing fasting glucose compared to the control commercial tea [82].

Gegen Qinlian Decoction (GQD)

Gegen Qinlian Decoction (GQD) is a traditional Chinese medicine obtained from the water extract of 4 herbs- Lobed Kudzuvine Root (*Puerariae lobatae* Radix; Gegen; *Pueraria lobata* (Willd.) Ohwi); Baical Skullcap Root (*Scutellariae* Radix; Huangqin; *Scutellaria baicalensis* Georgi); Golden Thread (*Coptidis* Rhizoma; Huanglian; *Coptis chinensis*); and Liquorice root (Glycyrrhizae Radix and Rhizoma Praeparata cum Melle; Zhigancao; *Glycyrrhiza uralensis*). Several clinical trials are available, which evaluated the efficacy of GQD in glycemic control on type 2 diabetic patients. All the trials reported the synergistic effect of GQD and metformin in improving blood sugar levels compared to that of metformin alone as a T2DM therapy [83]. It has been stated that glucose and energy metabolism is influenced by intestinal inflammation, since this condition changes gut flora [84, 85]. Gut flora are responsible for reducing serum glucose levels. Hence, GQD has been reported to have anti-inflammatory actions, which, in turn, improve blood glucose levels. However, GQD may mitigate the adverse effects observed in metformin therapy, like- diarrhoea, nausea, flatulence, indigestion, vomiting, abdominal discomfort, *etc* [83].

German Chamomile (*Matricaria chamomilla* L.)

German chamomile (*Matricaria chamomilla* L.) is composed of sesquiterpenes, flavonoids, coumarins, *etc*. Zemestani *et al.* enrolled 64 T2DM patients who were randomly divided to give either chamomile tea (3 g/150 mL hot water, thrice daily) immediately after meals or a water regimen for 8 weeks, in a single-blind, controlled study. They reported a significant reduction in glycosylated hemoglobin, serum insulin levels, homeostatic model assessment for insulin resistance, and serum malondialdehyde among the group taken chamomile tea compared to that of the control group [86].

Ginseng (*Panax quinquefolius*)

In 1995, Sotaniemi *et al.* carried out a double-blind, placebo-controlled trial on 36 NIDDM patients using either ginseng (100 or 200 mg) or placebo for 8 weeks. They revealed that ginseng reduced fasting blood glucose and HbA1c levels compared to the placebo [87]. Vuksan *et al.* (2000) conducted two studies on 10 healthy subjects and 9 T2DM patients administering 3 gm ginseng (*Panax quinquefolius*) or placebo capsules (composed of corn flour similar in quantity of carbohydrate and appearance to that of ginseng capsules), either 40 minutes before or together with a 25 gm oral glucose challenge. In healthy subjects, no changes were observed in postprandial glycemia between placebo and ginseng with the glucose challenge. However, significant reductions in postprandial glycemia were observed when ginseng was received 40 minutes before the glucose challenge. Ginseng capsules (taken before or together with the glucose challenge) significantly decreased postprandial glucose in T2DM patients [88].

GlucoSupreme Herbal

GlucoSupreme™ Herbal, a commercial polyherbal dietary supplement, is composed of cinnamon bark (*Cinnamomum cassia*), banaba leaf (*Lagerstroemia speciosa*), kudzu root (*Pueraria lobata*), fenugreek seed (*Trigonella foenum-graceum*), gymnema leaf (*Gymnema sylvestre*), American ginseng root (*Panax quinquefolius*), and berberine HCl derived from *Berberis aristata* bark. A multi-site, double-blinded, randomized controlled clinical trial hypothesized that this polyherbal dietary supplement is effective in restoring glycemic parameters to normal ranges in T2DM patients. They conducted the study on 40 participants with prediabetes giving either a daily oral GlucoSupreme™ Herbal or placebo for 12 weeks [89].

Green Tea *(Camellia sinensis)*

Green and black tea yield catechin and its derivatives, such as epigallocatechin, epigallocatechin gallate and epicatechin gallate [90]. In 2009, Nagao *et al.* performed a double-blind trial on T2DM patients who were not taking insulin therapy and randomly parted them to catechin group (*n* = 23) and control group (*n* = 20) for 12 weeks. The patients received one can of green tea (340 ml) of which catechin and caffeine contents were 582.8 mg and 72.3 mg in the catechin group, and 96.3 mg and 75.0 mg in the control group, respectively. Catechin did not significantly decrease FPG and HbA1c levels in the participants, but when consumed along with insulinotropic medications, it significantly reduced HbA1c level in T2DM patients. Moreover, the insulin level was significantly increased in the catechin group as well as compared to the control group without displaying any adverse-event during the study period and follow up for two-month [91].

Gymnema sylvestre

Gymnema sylvestre is widely used in controlling blood glucose, cholesterol and obesity in Ayurvedic medicine. The herb contains a mixture of saponins, known as gymnemic acid, which may be responsible for these activities. An uncontrolled trial used 800 mg of plant extract in a mixed population of 65 patients with type 1 and type 2 diabetes daily for 3 months. The trial showed significant fall in FBG and HbA1c levels without any adverse effect [92]. Kumar *et al.* (2010) reported a reduction in polyphagia, fatigue, blood glucose (fasting and post-prandial), and glycated hemoglobin using supplementation with 500 mg of the herb extract daily for 3 months, in an open label study [93]. In 1990, Baskaran *et al.* conducted a non-randomized open-label trial on 22 type 2 diabetic patients receiving either 400 mg of an ethanolic extract daily or their usual treatment for 18 to 20 months. They demonstrated that the extract significantly lower the blood glucose, glycosylated haemoglobin and glycosylated plasma proteins, which might lead to the reduction in usual drug dosage [94]. Shanmugasundaram *et al.* administered water-soluble extract of the leaves (400 mg/day) to 27 T1DM patients undergoing insulin therapy. Although the extract reduced insulin requirements as well as fasting blood glucose, HbAlc and glycosylated plasma protein levels in patients, there was no significant reduction in these parameters during follow up period after 10–12 months of the study [95].

Humulus lupulus L. (Hop)

The main ingredient of beer is Hops (*Humulus lupulus* L.), which contains isohumulone, isocohumulone and isoadhumulone. Obara *et al.* performed a double-blind, randomized trial to find out the effective dose of isohumulones in glycemic control. They enrolled 94 subjects with prediabetes and divided them into four groups giving either placebo capsules or test capsules comprising of 16 mg, 32 mg or 48 mg isohumulones daily for 12 weeks. After 4 weeks, fasting blood glucose was found to be reduced in the 32 mg and 48 mg dosage groups, as well as reduction in HbA1c level in the 16 mg group and after 8 weeks in the 32 mg and 48 mg groups [96].

Lignan from Flaxseed (*Linum usitatissimum*)

Flaxseed (*Linum usitatissimum*) is a rich source of dietary lignans. In 2006, 73 T2DM patients with mild hypercholesterolemia were allocated in a 12-week randomized, double-blind, placebo-controlled, cross-over trial receiving either flaxseed-derived lignan capsules (360 mg lignan daily) or placebo. The outcome of the trial showed that lignan supplement significantly reduced HbA_1c level compared to placebo [97].

Magnesium

Patients suffering from diabetes, glycosuria, ketoacidosis are found to have a common symptom like hypomagnesemia or excess urinary magnesium losses. A

1-month randomized, double-blind, placebo-controlled trial on 128 patients reported a significant reduction in serum fructosamine administering either placebo or 20.7 mmol MgO or 41.4 mmol elemental Mg daily [98]. In 1995, Eibl *et al.* also performed a double-blind, placebo-controlled trial on 40 T2DM patients with hypomagnesemia using 30 mmol oral magnesium daily. The findings of this trial demonstrated that oral magnesium replacement therapy improves hypomagnesemia in diabetic patients after a minimum treatment period of 3 months [99]. Decrease in FBG and increase in postprandial insulin were reported in a 4-week double-blind, randomized, crossover trial conducted on twelve aged subjects providing placebo or magnesium pidolate (4.5 g/d) [100]. Fifty poorly controlled T2DM patients were administered either 15 mmol Mg or placebo daily for 3 months in a trial by De Valk *et al.* and no change in FBG, HbA1C, and urine glucose were observed [101]. Paolisso *et al.* carried out two small trials (n=8 and n=9) using magnesium and revealed improvement in fasting plasma glucose and postprandial insulin levels [102, 103].

Mellissa officinalis L. (Lamiaceae) Based Product

In 2019, Nayebi *et al.* performed a double-blinded, controlled study using *Melissa officinalis* L. based product (MO) in 37 type 2 diabetic patients with dyslipidemia for 3 months. They randomly divided the patients into two groups and provided them with either MO (adding 150 mg of *R. damascena* aqueous extract to 350 mg of MO dried aqueous extract) or placebo (500 mg capsules twice) daily. The study reported that the preparation significantly reduced serum TG level in dyslipidemic diabetic patients [104].

Milk Thistle *(Silybum marianum)* (L.) Gaertn

Silybum marianum (L.) Gaertn, known as milk thistle, comprises many flavonolignans, of which silibinin (silybin) is the most significant. The seed extract of this plant is named as Silymarin, which is found to have antidiabetic effects in several studies. In 1997, Velussi *et al.* conducted a long-term trial to obseve the efficacy of silymarin in patients with type 2 diabetes and cirrhosis. The patients received 600 mg of silymarin daily for 12 months. In this study, significant reduction in HbA1c level, fasting plasma glucose (FPG), daily blood glucose average and glucosuria, daily insulin requirement, fasting insulin, as well as an increase in serum glutamic oxaloacetic transaminase (SGOT), serum glutamic pyruvic transaminase (SGPT) and HDL levels were observed in silymarin-treated group compared to the control group [105]. Huseini *et al.* carried out another short-term trial (4 months) with the same dosage form of silymarin as Velussi *et al.* and also found significant decrease in HbA1c, FPG, TC, LDL, TAG, SGOT and SGPT levels [106]. Silymarin was found to decrease

HbA1c, FPG, BMI and postprandial hyperglycemia when it is supplemented with glibenclamide in T2DM patients compared to control group receiving glibenclamide only [107]. Another 2-month study demonstrated a significant fall in HbA1c, LDL and total cholesterol levels, providing 200 mg of silymarin three times daily [108]. Mohammadi *et al.* (2013) reported significant reduction in insulin resistance and serum insulin levels compared with beginning as well as compared with the placebo group without significantly changing blood glucose and lipid profile [109].

Myrcia uniflora

Russo *et al.* (1990) conducted a double-blind, crossover trial to evaluate the efficacy of *Myrcia uniflora* infusion in glycemic control of T2DM patients. The trial divided allocated 10 healthy subjects and 18 Type II diabetic patients receiving placebo and infusion of 3 g leaves/day of *M. uniflora* for 56 days. *M. uniflora* infusion decreased plasma insulin levels in patients compared to the placebo group without changing plasma glucose levels or glycated hemoglobin [110].

Nigella sativa L.

A review of seven clinical trials indicated that *N. sativa* supplementation in type 2 diabetes patients significantly improved fasting blood glucose, HbA1c, total-cholesterol, and LDL level [111]. The hypoglycemic effect of *N. sativa* is hypothesized to be exerted due to the presence of thymoquinone, dithymoquinone, linoleic acid, and oleic acid, which might be responsible for stimulating pancreatic β-cells leading to insulin secretion, reducing hepatic gluconeogenesis, and inducing insulin sensitivity in peripheral tissue [112 - 118].

Onion *(Allium cepa)*

In 1975, Augusti *et al.* performed a randomized clinical trial in 6 non-diabetic subjects providing capsules containing allyl propyl disulphide extract from onion (*Allium cepa*) and reported significant improvement in the blood glucose levels and serum insulin level [119].

Opuntia streptacantha

Frati *et al.* carried out two controlled, short-term trials (*n*=14 and *n*=32) on subjects with NIDDM in 1990 and 1991. A significant decrease in fasting serum glucose and insulin levels was reported without any side effects in both trials [120, 121].

Pinus pinaster (French Maritime Pine)

Bark of French maritime pine (*Pinus pinaster* Aiton) yields a mixture of polyphenol commercially known as Pycnogenol. In 2004, Liu *et al.* observed the potency of pycnogenol performing a double-blind, placebo-controlled trial in patients with type 2 diabetes for 3 months. The patients received 100 mg pycnogenol daily. The study reported a significant decrease in HbA1c level during the first month of the trial period. Pycnogenol also significantly lowered FPG level especially in those who had FPG higher than 10 mmol/L [122]. Same investor group conducted another open labeled, controlled, dose-finding study among 30 T2DM patients using successive dosages of 50, 100, 200, and 300 mg pycnogenol in intervals of 3 weeks. After 1 month trial period, they observed maximum significant improvement in glycemic control at the dosage of 200 mg pycnogenol. Supplementation with pycnogenol also decreased endothelin-1, FPG, and LDL as well as albumin concentration in the urine [123]. 25 mg of pycnogenol was administered to patients with type 2 diabetes (5 times/day) in a trial, which showed a decrease in HbA1c significantly after the second and third month of the trial period compared to that of placebo [124].

Trifolium pratense (Red Clover)

Howes *et al.* demonstrated the beneficial effects of isoflavones from red clover (*Trifolium pretense*) on improving blood pressure and endothelial function in 16 women with postmenopausal type 2 diabetes using 50 mg of isoflavones daily in a randomized, double-blind, crossover trial for four weeks [125].

Resveratrol

Grape seeds and skin are the rich source of a polyphenol known as resveratrol. It is also extracted from knotweeds (*Polygonum cuspidatum*). In 2012, Bhatt *et al.* carried out an open-labeled, randomized, controlled trial using 250 mg resveratrol in T2DM patients treated with oral hypoglycemic medicines for 3 months. The resveratrol supplementation significantly reduced HbA1c, SBP and total cholesterol levels in patients [126]. Significant improvement was found in HbA1c and lipid profile in patients after 45 days receiving 1000 mg of resveratrol daily [127]. Another trial was conducted in 2014 by Witte *et al.* using 200 mg of resveratrol on cognitive function and glucose metabolism in overweight older adults. Resveratrol significantly reduced HbA1c as well as body fat levels after 26 weeks compared to placebo [128].

Scoparia dulcis L.

A 3-month randomized, crossover clinical trial showed a significant reduction in HbA1c level using herbal porridge prepared from *Scoparia dulcis* leaf extract 3 days/week in patients (n=35) with mild and moderate T2DM [129].

Semen Persical Decoction for Purgation with Addition (SPDPA)

Guangzhou University of Traditional Chinese Medicine (TCM) developed an antidiabetic formulation combining eight different herbs, known as Semen Persical decoction for purgation with addition (SPDPA). Xiong *et al.* (1995) revealed that SPDPA significantly reduced fasting blood glucose in a non-randomized, controlled clinical trial compared to the control group treated with glyburide (*n=148*) [130].

Soy Bean (*Glycin max*)

In 2005, Kim *et al.* performed a randomized, double-blind, placebo-controlled trial in T2DM patients (n=30), giving either 600 mg soybean-derived pinitol or placebo twice daily for 13 weeks. significant reduction in mean fasting plasma glucose, insulin, fructosamine, HbA_1c, HOMA-IR along with total cholesterol, LDL-cholesterol, the LDL/HDL-cholesterol ratio, systolic and diastolic blood pressure and rise in HDL-cholesterol levels were observed in pinitol treated group compared to the placebo group. This may be indicative to decreased risk of cardiovascular problems in type 2 diabetes mellitus [131].

Stevia rebaudiana

Stevia rebaudiana (Bertoni) contains steviol glycosides, which possess beneficial effects in glycemic control. A double-blind, placebo-controlled trial enrolled 76 individuals and randomly divided them into 3 groups: 16 Type 1 diabetic patients; 30 Type 2 diabetic patients and 30 subjects without diabetes and with normal/low-normal BP levels and providing them either 250 mg steviol glycoside (stevioside, thrice daily) or placebo for 3 months. No significant change was observed in glucose, HbA_1c levels as well as systolic BP, diastolic BP. However, significant improvement was found in systolic BP and glucose among the placebo Type 1 diabetics group without any side-effects [132].

Tibetan Medicine Herb Combination

Tibetan medicine is a traditional system that comprises of different healing concepts of Greece, China, India, Persia, as well as psychological, philosophical, and spiritual aspects of Buddhism [133]. An open level clinical trial evaluated a total of 200 Tibetan herb prescription of newly diagnosed or untreated T2DM patients on the basis of age, sex, personality, pulse, and urine characteristics. The treatment group was found to have lower fasting blood glucose, PPG, and glycated hemoglobin (GHb) levels compared to the control group at 12 and 24 weeks of trial period. Body weight, blood pressure or serum lipid levels remained unchanged in all groups [134].

Traditional Chinese Treatment (Multiple Herbal Combinations)

A controlled clinical trial was performed for the evaluation of antidiabetic effect of a Traditional Chinese Treatment (TCT) herbal preparation containing multiple herbs combination, including *Astragalus membranaceus, Coptis chinensis* and *Lonicera japonica*. Chinese Academy of Medical Science chose these three herbs on the basis of their safe and effective trial reports in treating diabetes along with a sulfonylurea, such as, glibenclamide (2.5 mg, 3 times daily). In 2013, Vray *et al.* conducted a double blind factorial design enrolling 216 tyoe 2 diabetic patients and randomly divided them into 4 groups: group A = placebo (P) TCT + P glibenclamide (n=56); group B = P TCT + verum glibenclamide (n=56); group C = verum TCT + P glibenclamide (n=50) and group D = verum TCT + verum glibenclamide (n=54). TCT showed significant synergistic improvement in controlling blood sugar levels with a sulfonylurea [135].

Tulsi/Holy Basil (*Ocimum sanctum*)

A 4-week, single-blind, controlled clinical trial reported decrease in fasting, postprandial glucose and urine glucose levels in 40 T2DM patients receiving 2.5 gm powder obtained from fresh leaves of *Ocimum sanctum* mixed in water [136].

Ulam Raja *(Cosmos caudatus)*

Ulam Raja (*Cosmos caudatus*), comprises ascorbic acid, quercetin, proanthocyanidin, chlorogenic acid and catechin, has beneficial effects in improving blood glucose levels. Cheng *et al.* enrolled 38 diabetic patients administering 15 g of *C. caudatus* daily and 39 diabetic patients receiving a normal diet in a single-center, randomized, and controlled two-arm parallel design clinical trial. Serum insulin, homeostatic model assessment-insulin resistance were significantly decreased as well as quantitative insulin sensitivity was increased in ulam-treated group compared to that of control group [137].

Vanadium

Vanadyl sulfate and sodium metavanadate are mostly used vanadium supplementation. Cohen *et al.* carried out a trial on six non-insulin-dependent diabetes mellitus (NIDDM) patients treated with/without sulfonylureas using

100mg/dL vanadil sulfate (VS) for 3 weeks. Improvement in hepatic and peripheral insulin sensitivity was observed in *VS* treated group compared to placebo group [138]. In 1996, Halberstam *et al.* performed another 3-week trial using the same dosage of *VS* in 7 NIDDM patients and 6 non-diabetics. This trial also reported improvement in both hepatic and skeletal muscle insulin sensitivity in diabetic patients, whereas, in non-diabetic group, insulin sensitivity was unchanged [139]. Decreased fasting blood glucose and hepatic insulin resistance were observed in 8 NIDDM patients providing 50 mg *VS* (two times/day) in a 4-week single-blind, placebo-controlled clinical trial conducted by Boden *et al.* [140]. Another two small, non-controlled, open-label trials also reported significant amelioration in glycemic control [141, 142]. Goldfine *et al.* (1995) enrolled 5 type 1 diabetic patients in the trial and demonstrated a reduction in insulin requirements after 2 weeks of vanadium supplementation [142]. Vanadium supplements are found to cause gastrointestinal troubles, like- flatulence, diarrhea, nausea, *etc.* whereas organically chelated compounds are hypothesized to cause less gastrointestinal discomfort [143].

Vitamin C

Vitamin C possesses significant free radical scavenging activities. In addition, diabetic patients were found to have 40–50% less vitamin C level in blood and tissues compared to non-diabetic individuals, which appears to be responsible for the maintenance of insulin action in humans [144 - 149]. In 1996, Ting *et al.* conducted a trial to investigate the efficacy of vitamin C in improving endothelium-dependent vasodilation. They enrolled 10 T2DM patients and 10 non-diabetic subjects as control using intra-arterial administration of vitamin C at a rate of 24 mg/min in association with 0.3–10 mg/min intraarterial infusion of methacholine (to assess endothelium-dependent vasodilation) and 0.3–10 mg/min nitroprusside and 10–300 mg/min verapamil (to assess endothelium-independent vasodilation). Infusion of vitamin C stimulated the vasodilating activity of methacholine, whereas vasodilation to nitroprusside and to verapamil remained unaffected by vitamin C. On the other hand, endothelium-dependent vasodilation was not affected by vitamin C infusion [150]. Paolisso *et al.* reported improvement in insulin action after infusing vitamin C (0.9 mmol/min) in ten healthy subjects and ten type 2 diabetic patients [151].

Vitamin E

Vitamin E possesses significant lipophilic antioxidant, protein glycation as well as insulin sensitivity and secretion activities. Four controlled trials reported beneficial effects of vitamin E supplementation in glycemic control in T2DM patients using doses ranging from 100-1600 mg/day for 2–4 months [152 - 155].

In contrast, serum glucose, fructosamine and HbA1c remained unchanged in a double-blind placebo-controlled crossover trial (n=53) [156]. 35 type 1 diabetic patients were found to have reduced protein glycosylation after 3 months of vitamin E (100 IU/day) supplementation [157].

Walnut Oil *(Juglan sregia* L.)

In 2017, a randomized, double-blind, placebo-controlled clinical trial was carried out on 100 hyperlipidemic T2DM patients receiving either 4 walnut oil capsules (1.25 cc) or 4 placebo capsules (1.25 cc distilled water) three times/day with meal for 90 days. This study showed improvement in lipid profiles of the patients after adding walnut oil in their daily meal [158].

Table 1. Clinical study reports of herbal plants, combined herbal preparations, extracts, bioactive compounds, functional foods, phytomedicines, traditional medicines and micronutrients for the evaluation of anti-diabetic actitivies.

Name of the Possible Phytoremedies Studied	Plant Part/ Phytoconstituents/ Materials used/composition	Study Design & Duration	Dosage and Groups	Outcomes	References
Aloe vera	Aloe gel	Non-randomized, single-blind, 2 parallel groups, uncontrolled on OHA for 42 days	T2DM patients (76), *A. vera* 80% juice; 1 tbsp BID with glibenclamide Control: Placebo juice	Decreased FBG No effects on liver/ kidney function	[29]
		Non-randomized, single-blind, 2 parallel groups, newly diagnosed patients for 42 days	T2DM patients (40), *A. vera* 80% juice: 1 tbsp BID Control: Placebo juice	Decreased FBG	[30]
		4-14 weeks	T2DM patients (5), dried sap of aloes, half a teaspoonful daily	Decreased FBG and HbA1c	[31]
		Randomized double-blind placebo controlled clinical trial for 2 months	T2DM patients (30) received aloe capsules (one 300 mg capsule every 12 hours by the oral route) combined with two 5 mg glyburide and two 500 mg metformin tablets daily and parallel group of thirty patients took the placebo capsules (orally every 12 hours)	Significantly lowered the fasting blood glucose, HbA1c, total cholesterol, and LDL-c levels compared to placebo	[32]
Alpha-lipoic Acid		Blinding unclear, 4 parallel groups, well-controlled on diet and/or OHA for 4 weeks	T2DM patients (74) received Alpha-lipoi- -acid 600 mg/d once *vs* 1200 mg/d twice *vs*. 1800 mg/d thrice Control: Placebo pill	Increased glucose uptake, decreased fasting insulin, improved insulin sensitivity, no change in FPG.	[33]
		Noncontrolled trial for 4 weeks	Lean (n= 10) and obese (n= 10) patients with type 2 diabetes received 600 mg α-lipoic-acid twice daily	Significantly increased fasting lactate and pyruvate levels	[34]

(Table 1) cont.....

Name of the Possible Phytoremedies Studied	Plant Part/ Phytoconstituents/ Materials used/composition	Study Design & Duration	Dosage and Groups	Outcomes	References
Artocarpus heterophyllus	Fresh mature leaves (200 g) of *A. heterophyllus* boiled with distilled water (1000 ml) for 3 h and the final volume reduced to 200 mL (1 mL equivalent to 1g of starting material).	Non-randomized, open-label, crossover, short-term metabolic trial	T2DM patients (10), 200 mL boiled decoction, prepared from 200g fresh leaves, single dose administered prior to GTT Control: 200 mL distilled water	Decreased PPG	[35]
Asteracanthus longifolia	Fresh whole plant material (100 g) of *A. longifolia* boiled with distilled water (1000 ml) for 3 h and the final volume reduced to 200 mL	Non-randomized, open-label, crossover, short-term metabolic trial	T2DM patients (10), 200 mL boiled decoction, prepared from 100g whole plant materials, single dose administration prior to GTT Control: 200 mL distilled water	Decreased PPG	[35]
Bell pepper *(Capsicum annuum* var. grossum) juice	Juice was prepared with 20g of bell pepper and 90 ml of water at room temperature	Randomized, controlled study for 4-consecutive days	Fifty T2DM diabetic subjects received 100-ml of bell pepper juice (twice/day) along with Yoga (integrated approach of Yoga therapy: IAYT) Control: only IAYT	Significantly reduced PPBG, SBP, pulse pressure (PP), rate pressure product (RPP) and double product (Do-P) compared with control group	[36]

(Table 1) cont.....

Name of the Possible Phytoremedies Studied	Plant Part/ Phytoconstituents/ Materials used/composition	Study Design & Duration	Dosage and Groups	Outcomes	References
Berberine	Berberine hydrochloride alkaloids obtained from *C. chinensis*	Study A: Randomized, controlled trial in newly diagnosed T2DM patients 13 weeks Study B: Uncontrolled study in poorly controlled T2DM patients 13 weeks	Study A: Berberine 1500 mg/d (18 patients) *vs.* metformin 1500 mg/d (18 patients) Study B: Oral Berberine 1500 mg/d (48 patients)	Significantly decreased HbA1c level, FPG, postprandial glucose, basal insulin and postprandial insulin in both groups HbA1c, FPG, PBG, basal insulin, HOMA-IR, fasting C-peptide and postprandial C-peptide were significantly improved.	[37]
	Berberine was extracted from rhizomes of *C. chinensis* with acidic water (0.3% H_2SO_4) soaking and chromatographic purification and had a purity 97% or greater.	Randomized, double-blind, placebo controlled, multicenter trial in T2DM patients with dyslipidemia 3 months	Berberine 1000 mg/d (57 patients) *vs.* placebo (49 patients)	HbA1c, FPG and PBG were significantly reduced in berberine group compared with the placebo group.	[38]
	Berberine (BBR), a nonprescription medicine in China	Randomized, controlled trial in type 2 diabetic patients 2 months	BBR 1000 mg/d (50 patients *vs.* metformin 1500 mg/d (26 patients) *vs.* rosiglitazone 4 mg/d (21 patients)	Improved insulin sensitivity Effective antihyperglycemic agent compared with metformin or rosiglitazone. Effectively managed glycemic profile in patients with hepatitis.	[39]
	Berberine (BBR), a nonprescription medicine in China	Randomized, double-blind, placebo controlled, multicenter trial in newly diagnosed T2DM patients 3 months	Berberine 1000 mg/d (30 patients) *vs.* placebo (30 patients)	Effective antihyperglycemic and antihyperglycemic agent.	[40]
	Berberine, Huashi Pharmaceuticals Shanghai, China	Randomized, open-label, controlled, multicenter clinical trial in T2DM patients with non-alcoholic fatty liver disease for 4 months	Berberine 1500 mg/d + life style intervention (LSI) (55 patients) *vs.* LSI (53 patients) *vs.* Pioglitazone 15 mg/d + LSI (47 patient)	Significantly decreased HbA_1c as well as other glycemic parameters in berberine plus LSI group compared with LSI only which was comparable with pioglitazone.	[41]
	Berberine, purchased from Guangdong, South China Pharmaceutical Group Co., Ltd.	Uncontrolled trial in T2DM patients for 2 months	Berberine 900 mg/d (30 patients)	Improved glycemic, lipidemic, and anthropometric parameters Significantly reduced inflammatory parameters- CPR, LPS and TNF-α	[42]
	Barberry fruit juice	Randomized clinical trial for 12 month	46 diabetic patients were randomly allocated to either the barberry juice (BJ) group (n=23) who consumed 200 mL of BJ daily, or the control group (n=23) with no intervention	Decreased the risk of cardiovascular diseases in patients with diabetes.	[43]

(Table 1) cont.....

Name of the Possible Phytoremedies Studied	Plant Part/ Phytoconstituents/ Materials used/composition	Study Design & Duration	Dosage and Groups	Outcomes	References
Berberol	*Berberis aristata* extract (588 mg) (standardized based on 85% berberine) and 105 mg *Silybum marianum* extract (standardized based on 60% flavonolignans)	Uncontrolled clinical trial in T2DM patients with suboptimal glycemic control for 3 months	Patients received berberol two times a day (22 patients)	Significantly reduced HbA1c level, basal insulin and HOMA-IR and increased insulin sensitivity.	[45]
		Randomized, single-blind, controlled clinical trial in T2DM patients for 4 months	A) Berberine 1000 mg/day (27 patients) B) Berberol two times a day (30 patients)	Both agents significantly reduced HbA1c and FPG; Berberol was more successful in reducing HbA1c level compared with berberine. Reduced SGOT and SGPT	[46]
		Uncontrolled trial in T2DM patients and hypercholesterolem-ic patients with statin-intolerance for 12 months	Berberol two times a day (45 patients: 15 patients treated with low-dose statins + 15 patients treated with ezetimibe + 15 untreated patients)	HbA1c and FPG were significantly reduced in all three mentioned groups without any serious side-effects. Significantly improved lipid profile	[47]

(Table 1) cont.....

Name of the Possible Phytoremedies Studied	Plant Part/ Phytoconstituents/ Materials used/composition	Study Design & Duration	Dosage and Groups	Outcomes	References
Bitter gourd/Bitter melon *(Momordica charantia)* (V-insulin)	Fruit juice (Polypeptide-P, vicine, momordin, momordicin, charantin momorcharaside A and B, momorcharin A and B are phytoconstituents of bitter groud)	Non-randomized, open-label, crossover, short-term metabolic trial, newly diagnosed patients	Type 2 patients (18) received *M. charantia* Juice, homemade preparation (dose unspecified), single experimental dose prior to GTT control: Distilled water	Decreased PPG	[49]
	Suspension of vegetable insulin (purified protein extract: 1.8 mg per 40 units) administered by subcutaneous or the intra- muscular route	Non-randomized, blinding unclear, 2 parallel groups, short-term metabolic trial, all on insulin/OHA stopped during study	9 DM (6 Type 1, 3 Type 2), *M. charantia* vegetable insulin (purified protein extract), single severity dependent experimental dose (subcutaneous) Control: Placebo injection (unspecified)	Decreased FBG. No hyper-sensitivity reaction.	[50]
		Multicenter, randomized, double-blind, active-control trial for 4-week	120 type 2 diabetic patients, were randomized into 4 groups to receive bitter melon 500 mg/day, 1000 mg/day, and 2000 mg/day or metformin 1000 mg/day	Significantly reduced fructosamine levels from baseline among patients with type 2 diabetes who received bitter melon 2000 mg/day	[51]
	To mask the bitter taste, 0.75g alpha-cyclodextrin mixed with 2% lemon peel oil, 75 mg beta-cyclodextrin, 15 mg steviol glyscoside, and 0.75 g cucumber powder were added to the bitter gourd powder	Randomized placebo-controlled, single blinded clinical trial for 8 weeks	Prediabetic subjects (52) divided into an AB-BA sequence, received daily dosage of bitter gourd powder: 2.5 g, placebo received 3.25 g cucumber powder "Group 1" (AB) started with bitter gourd supplementation, followed by placebo after a washout period of four weeks. "Group 2" (BA) started with placebo followed by bitter gourd supplementation with the same washout period in between	Lowered elevated fasting plasma glucose in prediabetic subjects. No effect on insulin or HbA1c. Some mild adverse effects after bitter gourd consumption were reported, *e.g.* flatulence, loose stools, mild diarrhea, headache, nausea, and vomiting, but no hypoglycemia	[52]

(Table 1) cont.....

Name of the Possible Phytoremedies Studied	Plant Part/ Phytoconstituents/ Materials used/composition	Study Design & Duration	Dosage and Groups	Outcomes	References
Carnitine		Blinding unclear, crossover, short-term metabolic clinical trial	T2DM diabetic patients (9) received carnitine: 1.7 mmol/min, constant intravenous infusion with euglycemic hyperinsulinemic clamp Control: Saline infusion	Increased glucose uptake and insulin sensitivity.	[53]
	Acetyl-L Carnitine	Double-blind, Crossover, short-term metabolic trial, on diet, OHA, and/or insulin (switched to insulin during study)	Type 2 diabetic patients (18) received intravenous infusion of acetyl-L-carnitine: 0.025 mg/kg/min *vs* 0.1 mg/kg/min, constant infusion during euglycemic hyperinsulinemic clamp Control: Saline infusion	Increased glucose uptake, glucose storage; decreased serum insulin. No change in glucose or lipid oxidation.	[54]
	L-Carnitine	Blinding unclear, crossover, short-term metabolic trial, on diet and OHA (switched to insulin during study)	Type 2 diabetic patients (15) received L-Carnitine: 0.28 mol/kg bw/min, simultaneous infusion with euglycemic hyperinsulinemic clamp Control: Saline infusion	Increased glucose uptake, glucose oxidation, glucose storage, insulin sensitivity.	[55]
Caucasian whortleberry (*Vaccinium arctostaphylos* L.) and Cinnamon		Randomized triple-blinded, placebo controlled clinical trial for 2 years	Thirty patients each were randomly allocated to receive cinnamon (1000 mg/day) or Caucasian whortleberry (1000 mg/day), with the remaining 45 patients being allocated to the placebo group and being treated with starch (1000 mg/day) for 3 months	Significant reduction of FBG, 2-h PPG, serum insulin, HbA1c levels, and HOMA-IR scores.	[56]
Celery (*Apium graveolens* L.)	Leaf	Randomized control trials for 12 days	Elderly pre-diabetics (16) treated with 250 mg celery, given 3 times/day, Placebo group (250 mg lactose, magnesium stearate and aerosil)	Effectively reduced blood glucose levels, but there was a lack of association between blood glucose levels and plasma insulin levels.	[57]

(Table 1) cont.....

Name of the Possible Phytoremedies Studied	Plant Part/ Phytoconstituents/ Materials used/composition	Study Design & Duration	Dosage and Groups	Outcomes	References
Chromium	Chromium picolinate	Double-blind, Crossover clinical study for 2 months	T2DM patients (30) on diet, OHA, and/or insulin received chromium picolinate: 200 g/d (unspecified preparation); Control: Placebo pill	No change in FBG and HbA1c. No side-effect.	[58]
	Chromium picolinate	Double-blind, 3 parallel groups, on diet, OHA, and/or TCM meds for 8 weeks	T2DM patients (180) received chromium picolinate: 200 g/d *vs* 1000 g/d Control: Matched placebo pill	Decreased HbA1c, fasting and postprandial insulin (both doses); decreased FBG and PPG (high dose) No side-effect	[59]
	Chromium picolinate	Double-blind, 2 parallel groups clinical trials for 8 months	Obese nondiabetic patients (29) at risk for Type 2 diabetes mellitus received chromium picolinate: 1000 µg/d (preparation unspecified) Control: Placebo	Increased insulin sensitivity but no change in FPG, PPG, HbA1c, fructosamine, weight. Decreased insulin level.	[60]
	Organic chromium (Brewer's yeast capsule) *vs* Inorganic chromium	Double-blind, multiple crossover clinical study for 8 weeks	T2DM patients (78) on diet, OHA, and/or insulin received organic chromium (Brewer's yeast capsule 23.3 g Cr/day) *vs* inorganic chromium (CrCl$_3$ capsule 200g Cr/day) Control: Torula yeast capsule	Decreased FPG, PPG, fructosamine (both Cr supplement types), no change in BMI No side-effect	[61]
	Chromium-rich yeast	Double-blind, 2 parallel groups clinical study for 6 months	26 elderly with impaired glucose tolerance received chromium-rich yeast: 160 µg/d in 4 pellets (unspecified preparation) Control: Identical placebo pellets	No change in FBG, PPG, postprandial insulin, HbA1c, C-peptide and BMI	[62]
	Chromium Chloride	Double-blind, Crossover clinical study for 4 weeks	Patients with impaired glucose tolerance (8) received chromium chloride: 200 µg/d (preparation unspecified) Control: Placebo tablet	Decreased PPG, postprandial insulin and glucagon	[63]
	Chromium chloride	Blinding unclear, 2 parallel groups for 7–16 months clinical trials	T2DM patients (25) with atherosclerotic disease on diet and/or OHA received chromium chloride: 250 µg/d in syrup (preparation unspecified) Control: Placebo supplement in syrup	Chromium supplementation for periods of up to 16 months produced no initial or long-term changes in fasting blood glucose concentrations in diabetic or nondiabetic subjects.	[64]

(Table 1) cont.....

Name of the Possible Phytoremedies Studied	Plant Part/ Phytoconstituents/ Materials used/composition	Study Design & Duration	Dosage and Groups	Outcomes	References
	Chromium, Zinc combination	Double-blind; 4 parallel groups, well-controlled on diet, OHA, and/or insulin for 6 months	110 T2DM patients received chromium pidolate 400 g/d *vs.* Zinc gluconate 30 mg/d *vs.* Zn/Cr combination *vs.* placebo pill	Decreased plasma thiobarbituric acid reactive substances (TBARS); no change in FPG, HgbA1C, insulin, weight, BMI (in all supplement groups)	[65]
Cinnamon *(Cinnamomum zeylanicum)*	Cinnamon powder (*Cinnamomum zeylanicum*) or extract containing cinnamaldehyde as bioactive compound	Meta-analysis of 10 randomized clinical trials for 4-18 weeks study periods	Cinnamon extract or powder with doses 120 mg/day - 6g/day among 543 patients	Reduced FPG (-24.59 mg/dL), TC (-15.60 mg/dL), LDL-c (-9.42 mg/dL), and TG (-29.59 mg/dL). Increased HDL-c (1.66 mg/dL) and non-significant reduction of HbA1c (–0.16%)	[66]
	One cinnamon capsule contained 112 mg of the aqueous cinnamon extract, corresponding to 1 g of cinnamon	Double-blind design for 4 month	79 patients with diagnosed diabetes mellitus type 2 not on insulin therapy but treated with oral antidiabetics or diet were randomly assigned to take either a cinnamon extract or a placebo capsule (microcrystalline cellulose) three times daily	Significantly reduced blood glucose level in the cinnamon group than in the placebo group No adverse effect	[67]
Coccinia indica	Freeze-dried powder from fresh leaves (powder contained guar gum, pectin and pectin fibres, mucilaginous fibre)	Double-blind, 2 parallel groups, uncontrolled or untreated T2DM patients 6 weeks	T2DM patients (32) *Coccinia indica* leaf powder 1800 mg/d as tablets Control: Placebo tablet	Decreased FBG and PPG No side effect, no effect on liver or kidney functions	[68]
	Dried pellets from fresh leaves	Non-randomized, open-label, 3 parallel groups 12 weeks	T2DM patients (70), *C. indica* 6g/day Control: treatment with OHA	Decreased FBG, PPG similar to OHA	[69]
	Dried extract of leaves	Open-label trial 6 weeks	Diabetes patients (30), *C. indica* 500 mg/kg (body weight)	*C. indica* act like insulin, correcting the elevated enzymes G-6-p (ase), LDH in glycolytic pathway and restore the LPL activity in lypolytic pathway with the control of hyperglycemia in diabetes.	[70]
Corn bran (Zea species)	Water-soluble hemicellulose extracted from corn bran (corn bran hemicelluloses: CBH)	Controlled trial in obese and non-obese patients for 6 months	CBH 10000 mg/d (20 obese, 8 nonobese) *vs* 10 healthy subjects (control)	Long-term supplementation with CBH decreased HbA1c significantly in the obese patients, while the fasting glucose level decreased in all three groups, although not significantly.	[71]

(Table 1) cont.....

Name of the Possible Phytoremedies Studied	Plant Part/ Phytoconstituents/ Materials used/composition	Study Design & Duration	Dosage and Groups	Outcomes	References
Curcumin from *Curcuma longa* (Turmeric)	Two capsules containing curcumin 150 mg twice daily	Randomized, placebo-controlled, parallel-group trial in T2DM patients for 2 months	Curcumin 300 mg/d (23 patients) *vs.* atorvastatin 10 mg/d (23 patents) *vs.* placebo (21 patients)	HbA1c level and lipid profile were not significantly changed in curcumin-treated group.	[72]
	Curcuminoids (botanical extracts isolated from the rhizome of turmeric)	Randomized, double-blind, placebo controlled trial in T2DM patients for 3 months	Curcuminoid 300 mg/d (50 patients) *vs.* placebo (50 patients)	HbA1c was significantly reduced in curcumin-treated group compared with the placebo group. Also, remarkable decrease in triacylglycerol (TAG) and free fatty acid (FFA) level	[73]
	Nano-curcumin is a registered curcumin product (SinaCurcumin®) for oral use. Each soft gel of Nano-curcumin contains 80 mg of curcumin in the form of nano-micelle.	Randomized, double blind, placebo controlled, add-on clinical trial in T2DM patients for 3 months	Nano-curcumin (as nano-micelle) 80 mg/d (3513 patients) *vs.* placebo (3145 patients)	Significant reduction in HbA1c level as well as TAG, TC and BMI of curcumin treated group	[74]
Curcuminoids (Turmeric) plus piperine	5 mg piperine was added to each 500 mg curcuminoids capsule	Randomized double-blind placebo controlled trial for 12 weeks	Subjects with T2D (n=118) were assigned to curcuminoids (1000 mg/day plus piperine 10 mg/day) Control: placebo plus standard of care for T2D	Curcuminoids supplementation reduced serum levels of atherogenic lipid indices including non-HDL-C and lipoprotein (a) (Lp(a))	[75]
Dia-Best™ (a herbal formulation)	Cinnamon bark (*Cinnamomum zeylanicum*), Fenugreek seed (*Trigonella foenum-graceum*), *Nigella sativa* seed, Oat, *Ganoderma lucidum*, and Bitter gourd powder	Single blind prospective intervention study for 60 days	30 uncontrolled type 2 diabetes patients receiving oral medications and/or insulin, were orally admistered with 1 sachet of powder (3g powder/sachet) of DiabCure in the morning 20 minutes before breakfast and at night 1 hour before sleep	Significantly reduced fasting blood glucose levels, HbA1c, post-prandial blood glucose levels, total serum cholesterol, low density lipoprotein (LDL-c), and triglyceride (TG) levels No major adverse-effect	[76]

(Table 1) cont.....

Name of the Possible Phytoremedies Studied	Plant Part/ Phytoconstituents/ Materials used/composition	Study Design & Duration	Dosage and Groups	Outcomes	References
Fenugreek *(Trigonella foenum-graecum)*	Seeds as condiment	i) Metabolic study; crossover, diet and OHA (dose decreased 20% during study) for 10 days ii) Metabolic, crossover study for 20 days	i) T2DM patients (15), defatted fenugreek seed powder: 100 g/day in unleavened bread Control: Protein isolate from groundnut ii) Type 2 diabetic patients (5) with diet and OHA (dose decreased 20% during study) administered with defatted fenugreek seed powder: 100 g/day in unleavened bread Control: Protein isolate from groundnut	i) The mean fasting blood glucose level decreased from 179 ± 24 mg/dl to 137 + 20.2 mg/dl after 10 days of fenugreek diet. Serum insulin levels and integrated insulin area were also significantly lower after fenugreek diet as compared to control diet (P~0.05). ii) The mean fasting blood glucose level decreased after ingestion of fenugreek. These reductions were found to be statistically significant (P<0.05). There was an improvement in glucose tolerance and significant reduction in 24 hr urinary glucose excretion, serum cholesterol and triglyceride levels (P < 0.05).	[77]
	Defatted fenugreek seed powder	Randomized, blinding unclear, crossover study with diet and insulin (dose decreased during study) for 10 days	Treated: T1DM patients (10), defatted fenugreek seed powder: 100 g/d in unleavened bread Control: No treatment	Decreased FBG, PPG, urine glucose No change body weight, and insulin.	[78]
	The defatted meat, gum isolate and degummed material from seeds and fresh leaves of fenugreek	Randomized, crossover study for 21 days	Healthy volunteers (*n*=38), six protocols involved the acute administration (single dose of 25 g of seeds, 5 g of gum isolate and 150 g of leaves) of whole fenugreek seeds, defatted fenugreek seeds, gum isolate, degummed fenugreek seeds, cooked fenugreek seeds and cooked fenugreek leaves	Whole raw seeds, extracted seed powder, gum isolate of seeds, and cooked whole seeds seemed to decrease postprandial glucose levels, whereas degummed seeds and cooked leaves did not.	[79]
	Fenugreek seed powder	Non-randomized, open-label, crossover, short-term metabolic trial for 6 months	T2DM patients (21); Fenugreek seed powder: 15 g in water, single experimental dose with meal tolerance test Control: No treatment	Decreased PPG, No change in plasma insulin. No side-effects	[80]
	TFGs capsules (0.35 g/pill, each gram of powder equals to 16 g of crude drug)	Randomized, double-blind, placebo paralleled trial in T2DM patients for 3 months	Total saponins: Three times a day, each time 6 capsule (0.35 g/pill) (46 patients) *vs* placebo three times a day, each time 6 capsules (23 patients)	Remarkable decrease in FBG, 2-h post-prandial blood glucose and HbA1c levels in treated group as compared to control group.	[81]
Ficus carica (Fig leaves)	Leaves decoction	Open-label, crossover with diet and insulin 4 weeks	T1DM patients (10), decoction of fig leaves tea, 13 g/d Control: Bitter commercial tea blend	Decreased PPG and insulin requirement. No change in FPG, C-peptide, HgbA1c No side effects.	[82]

(Table 1) cont.....

Name of the Possible Phytoremedies Studied	Plant Part/ Phytoconstituents/ Materials used/composition	Study Design & Duration	Dosage and Groups	Outcomes	References
Gegen Qinlian Decoction (GQD)	Water extracts of mainly 4 herbs comprised of Lobed Kudzuvine Root (*Puerariae Lobatae* Radix; Gegen; *Pueraria lobata* (Willd.) *Ohwi* (*Fabaceae*); Baical Skullcap Root (*Scutellariae* Radix; Huangqin; *Scutellaria baicalensis* Georgi); Golden Thread (*Coptidis* Rhizoma; Huanglian; *Coptis chinensis*); and Liquorice root (Glycyrrhizae Radix and Rhizoma Praeparata cum Melle; Zhigancao; *Glycyrrhiza uralensis*)	Randomized control clinical trials for 8 weeks	Control group was provided 0.5~2.5 g metformin/day over two doses and experimental groups received the same dosage of metformin plus GQD	Highly effective adjunct to metformin as a treatment for type 2 diabetes.	[83]
German chamomile (*Matricaria chamomilla* L.)	Chamomile was obtained as homogenous chamomile tea bags (finished product, 3g) from the Iranian Institute of medicinal plants, Karaj Iran	single-blind, randomized, controlled clinical trial for 8 weeks	64 subjects, (n=32) consumed chamomile tea (3 g/150 mL hot water) 3 times per day. The control group (n =32) followed a water regimen.	Short term intake of chamomile tea has beneficial effects on glycemic control and antioxidant status in patients with T2DM.	[86]
Ginseng (Unspecified)	Ginseng tablet (Dansk Droge, Copenhagen) (Ginseng contains phytochemicals: ginsenosides or panaxosides phytochemicals)	Double-blind, 3 parallel groups, newly diagnosed T2DM patients 8 weeks	T2DM (36), Ginseng 100 mg/d *vs*. 200 mg/d Control: Placebo tablet	Decreased FBG and HbA1c (200 mg). No change in BG and insulin levels.	[87]
Ginseng (*Panax quinquefolius*)	Gelatin capsules containing 3 g of American, Ontario-grown ginseng root (Ginseng contains phytochemicals: ginsenosides or panaxosides phytochemicals)	Single-blind, multiple crossover, short-term metabolic trial with diet and/or OHA	Nondiabetic patients (10), Ground root of American ginseng; 3 g *vs* 6 g *vs* 9 g capsules, single experimental dose at varying times prior to OGTT Control: Identical placebo capsule containing cornflour	Decreased PPG (all doses), no difference between doses or administration times. No side-effect	[88]
		Single-blind, multiple crossover, short-term metabolic trial, well controlled on diet and/or OHA	T2DM patients (9), ground root of American ginseng: 3 g capsule, single experimental dose at varying times prior to OGTT Control: Identical placebo capsule containing cornflour	Significantly decreased PPG Mild insomnia was observed in one of the nine patients.	[88]

(Table 1) cont.....

Name of the Possible Phytoremedies Studied	Plant Part/ Phytoconstituents/ Materials used/composition	Study Design & Duration	Dosage and Groups	Outcomes	References
GlucoSupreme Herbal	Cinnamon bark (*Cinnamomum cassia*), banaba leaf (*Lagerstroemia speciosa* standardized to 1% corosolic acid), kudzu root (*Pueraria lobata* standardized to 40% isoflavones), fenugreek seed (*Trigonella foenum-graceum* standardized to 60% saponins), gymnema leaf (*Gymnema sylvestre* standardized to 25% gymnemic acid), American ginseng root (*Panax quinquefolius* standardized to 5% ginsenosides), and berberine HCl derived from bark (*Berberis aristata*)	Randomized, double-blinded, placebo controlled clinical trial with prediabetes subjects for 12 weeks	Study subjects: 40 prediabetic patients, received four GlucoSupreme herbal capsules Control: Placebo	May restore glycemic parameters to normal ranges, irrespective of broad changes in diet or physical activity.	[89]
Green tea (*Camellia sinensis*)	The control and catechin-rich beverages were prepared by the addition of green tea extract to brewed green tea. The catechin content in one can (340 ml) was 582.8 mg (caffeine 72.3 mg) in the catechin-rich beverage, and 96.3 mg (caffeine 75 mg) in the control beverage.	Randomized, double-blind, controlled parallel group, multicenter trial in T2DM patients for 3 months	Catechins 582.8 mg/d (23 patients) *vs.* catechins 96.3 mg/d (control, 20 patients)	Catechin-rich beverage might have impacts in the prevention of obesity; in the recovery of insulin-secretory ability; and, to maintain low HbA1c levels in type 2 diabetic patients	[91]

(Table 1) cont.....

Name of the Possible Phytoremedies Studied	Plant Part/ Phytoconstituents/ Materials used/composition	Study Design & Duration	Dosage and Groups	Outcomes	References
Gymnema sylvestre (Gurmar)	*G. sylvestre* extract	Open-label, uncontrolled trial for 3 months	65 patients with T1DM and T2DM given oral dose of 800 mg daily of *G. sylvestre* extract	FBG and HbA1c were reduced.	[92]
	GS in the form of capsules containing extracts of the leaves	Open-label study for 3 months	A control group (N=19) and an experimental group (N=39). Oral dose of GS 500 mg of herbal extract.	Reduced polyphagia, fatigue, blood glucose (fasting and postprandial), and HbA1c in comparison to the control group.	[93]
	Water-soluble acidic fraction of an ethanol extract of the leaves of *G. sylvestre*	Non-randomized, open-label, 2 parallel groups, all on OHA for 18–20 months	T2DM patients (22), ethanolic extract *of G. sylvestre:* 400 mg/d in capsule Control: No treatment	Decreased FBG, HbA1c, glycosylated plasma protein, urine glucose and conventional medication but increase in serum insulin level.	[94]
		Non-randomized, open-label, 2 parallel groups, all patients were on insulin treatment received gymnema for 10-12 months	T1DM patients (27), *G. sylvestre* extract, GS_4; 400 mg/d capsule Control: No treatment	Decreased FBG, HbA1c, glycosylated plasma protein, urine glucose and insulin requirement but increase in C-peptide. No side-effect	[95]
Humulus lupulus L. (Hop)	A soft capsule containing isomerized hop extract. One test capsule contained about 8 mg of isohumulones (isohumulone, isocohumulone, iso-adhumulone ratio, 49:35:16; respectively).	Randomized double-blind placeb ocontrolled trial in prediabetic patients for 12 weeks	94 patients, Isohumulone group 1: 16 mg/d (22 patients); group 2: 32 mg/d (20 patients); group 3: 48 mg/d (21 patients) *vs* placebo (21 patients)	Fasting blood glucose was decreased in patients receiving 32 mg and 48 mg after 4 weeks, but no change observed placebo group. HbA1c was also significantly decreased after 4 weeks in 16 mg group and after 8 weeks in 32 mg and 48 mg groups.	[96]
Lignan from Flax seed *(Linum usitatissimum)*	Lignin capsules (0.6 g/capsule)	Randomized, double-blind, placebo controlled, crossover trial in T2DM patients for 3 months	T2DM patients (73); Flaxseed-derived lignan: 360 mg/d (68 patients) *vs* placebo (same population)	Significantly reduced HbA_{1c} compared to placebo; no significant changes in fasting glucose and insulin concentration, insulin resistance and blood lipid profiles. Urinary excretion of lignan metabolites (enterodiol and enterolactone) was significantly higher after the lignan supplement intervention compared to baseline	[97]

(Table 1) cont.....

Name of the Possible Phytoremedies Studied	Plant Part/ Phytoconstituents/ Materials used/composition	Study Design & Duration	Dosage and Groups	Outcomes	References
Magnesium (Mg)	Magnesium oxide	Double-blind, 3 parallel groups, poorly controlled (with neuropathy and CAD) on diet and/or OHA for 30 days	T2DM patients (128) received magnesium oxide: 20.7 mmol/d *vs* 41.4 mmol/d elemental Mg Control: Placebo pill	Decreased fructosamine (higher dose); no change in FBG, HbA1c and BMI. No side-effect	[98]
	Magnesium citrate	Double-blind, 2 parallel groups, well controlled on diet and OHA for 3 months	T2DM patients (40) with Hypomagnesemia, magnesium citrate: 30 mmol/d Control: Placebo pill	No change in HbA1C, FBG, PPG and insulin	[99]
	Magnesium pidolate	Double-blind, randomized, crossover study for 4 weeks	12 nondiabetic (elderly with insulin resistance) received magnesium pidolate: 4.5g /d chronic magnesium administration (CMA) Control: Placebo pill	Decreased FBG, increased postprandial insulin, glucose uptake, and glucose oxidation; unclear C-peptide.	[100]
	Magnesium aspartate HCl	Blinding unclear, 2 parallel groups all on diet and insulin for 3 months clinical study	T2DM patients (50) received magnesium aspartate HCl: 15 mmol/d Control: Placebo	No change in FBG, HbA1c, urine glucose. No side-effect	[101]
	Magnesium pidolate	Double-blind, crossover study for 4 weeks	9 T2DM patients, elderly, nonobese on diet alone received magnesium pidolate: 4.5 g/d Control: Placebo	Improved insulin sensitivity and glucose oxidation during clamp. No change in FPG, C-peptide, glucagon and body weight.	[102]
	Chronic magnesium administration	Open-label, Crossover study on diet and OHA (diet alone during study) for 4 weeks	T2DM patients (8) received chronic magnesium administration: 2 mg/d Control: Placebo pill	Decreased FPG and increased postprandial insulin levels.	[103]
Mellissa officinalis L. (Lamiaceae) based product (in combination with *Rosa damascena* Mill.)	Aerial parts of *M. officinalis* (MO) and flowers of *R. damascena*	Randomized double-blinded controlled study for 3 months	T2DM patients (37) received capsules prepared by adding 150 mg of *R. damascena* aqueous extract to 350 mg of MO dried aqueous extract. The placebo capsules were filled by 500 mg of maize starch	Safe and beneficial in decreasing the serum TG level in dyslipidemic diabetic patients.	[104]

(Table 1) cont.....

Name of the Possible Phytoremedies Studied	Plant Part/ Phytoconstituents/ Materials used/composition	Study Design & Duration	Dosage and Groups	Outcomes	References
Milk thistle *(Silybum marianum)*	Legalon® from IBI Lorenzini, Milan, Italy (Phytoconsituent: Silymarin)	Randomized, open-label, controlled study in T2DM patients with cirrhosis for 12 months	Silymarin 600 mg/d (30 patients) *vs* untreated (30 patients)	Significant decrease in HbA1c level, FPG, daily blood glucose average and glucosuria, daily insulin requirement average and fasting insulin level of silymarin-treated group.	[105]
	200 mg silymarin tablet	Randomized, double-blind, placebo controlled, clinical trial in T2DM patients for 4 months	Silymarin 600 mg/d (25 patients) *vs* placebo (26 patients)	HbA1c, FPG, TC, LDL, TAG, SGOT and SGPT levels were significantly decreased compared to baseline levels.	[106]
	Silymarin capsule	Randomized, double-blind, placebo controlled multicenter, clinical trial in T2DM patients for 4 months	Silymarin 200 mg/d and glibenclamide 10 mg/d (18 patients) *vs* placebo and glibenclamide 10 mg/d (20 patients) *vs* control group with only glibenclamide 10 mg/d (21 patients)	Significantly reduced HbA1c, FPG and BMI, postprandial hyperglycemia in silymarin-treated group.	[107]
	Silymarin tablet (200 mg)	Randomized, double-blind, placebo controlled clinical trial in T2DM patients for 2 months	Silymarin 600 mg/d (30 patients) *vs* placebo (30 patients)	HbA1c and other glycemic parameters as well as LDL and total cholesterol were significantly decreased.	[108]
	Silymarin capsules (140 mg)	Randomized, placebo-controlled trial in healthy obese cases with family history of T2DM for 3 months	Silymarin 280 mg/d (30 cases) *vs* placebo (30 cases)	Significant reduction in insulin resistance and serum insulin levels compared with beginning as well as compared with placebo group without significantly changing blood glucose and lipid profile.	[109]
Myrcia uniflora	Infusion of leaves	Double-blind, crossover, patients with diet and/or OHA for 8 weeks	T2DM patients (18), *M.uniflora* tea: 3g/d Control: Placebo herb tea (sape, *Imperata brasiliensis*)	Plasma insulin levels in the diabetic group were lower after *M. uniflora* than after placebo	[110]
Nigella sativa	Nigella powder or extract (Thymoquinone is the main bioactive compound)	Meta-analysis of 7 clinical trials	*Nigella sativa* extracts or powders were supplemented to type 2 diabetes patients	Significantly reduced FBS, HbA1c, TC and LDL-c Insignificant reduction of TG and HDL-c	[111]
Onion *(Allium cepa)*	Allylpropyl disulphide (APDS) isolated from fresh onion is enclosed in a gelatin capsule	Randomized control trial	nondiabetic volunteers (*n*=6), APDS in gelatin capsule (0.125 g/50 kg) body weight	Significant fall in the blood glucose and significant rise in serum insulin level	[119]

(Table 1) cont.....

Name of the Possible Phytoremedies Studied	Plant Part/ Phytoconstituents/ Materials used/composition	Study Design & Duration	Dosage and Groups	Outcomes	References
Opuntia streptacantha (Nopal)	Stem powder (contains Fiber and pectin)	Open-label, Crossover, short-term metabolic trial with diet and/or OHA (diet alone during study)	T2DM patients(14), grilled nopal stems: 500 g single experimental dose Control: 400 ml H_2O	Significantly decreased glucose and serum insulin.	[120]
		Non-randomized, open-label, crossover, short-term metabolic trial; OHA stopped during study	T2DM patients (32), fresh nopal stems, broiled: 500 g crude weight; single experimental dose Control: Water, broiled zucchini squash	Significantly decreased glucose and serum insulin.	[121]
Pinus pinaster (French maritime Pine)	Pycnogenol, extract of bark from the French maritime pine, *P. pinaster*, represents a concentrate of water-soluble polyphenols	Randomized, double-blind, placebo controlled, parallel group, multicenter study in T2DM patients for 3 months	Pycnogenol 100 mg/d (34 patients) *vs* placebo (43 patients)	HbA1c level was significantly reduced during the first month of the trial. FPG was significantly reduced in Pycnogenol group especially in patients with a baseline FPG higher than 10 mmol/L.	[122]
		Open, controlled, dose-finding study in T2DM patients for 4 months	Pycnogenol 200 mg/d or 300 mg/d (30 patients)	Pycnogenol (200 mg) was determined as the maximum glucose lowering dose. No further reduction effect in doses over 300 mg was observed.	[123]
		Randomized, double-blind, placebo controlled parallel-group trial in T2DM patients for 3 months	Pycnogenol 125 mg/d (24 patients) *vs* placebo (24 patients)	HbA1c was reduced.	[124]
Trifolium pratense (Red clover)	Dietary supplementation with isoflavones from red clover (approximately 50 mg/day)	Randomized double-blind, placebo controlled, crossover trial in postmenopausal T2DM patients for 4 weeks	Postmenopausal type 2 diabetics treated with ≈50 mg/d (16 patients) *vs* placebo (same population)	Isoflavone supplementation from red clover may favourably influence blood pressure and endothelial function in postmenopausal type 2 diabetic women.	[125]
Resveratrol	Oral supplementation of resveratrol	Randomized, open-label, controlled trial in T2DM patients for 3 months	Resveratrol 250 mg/d (28 patients) *vs* control group (29 patients received only oral antihyperglycemic drugs)	Significant decrease in HbA1c level, SBP and total cholesterol in T2DM patients with resveratrol supplementation under oral antihyperglycemic therapy.	[126]
		Randomized, double-blind, placebo controlled, parallel clinical trial in T2DM patients for 45 days	Resveratrol 1000 mg/d (33 patients) *vs* placebo (31 patients)	Significant reduction in HbA1c level after 45 days of treatment. Glycemic and lipid profile parameters of patients were also improved comparing to baseline levels.	[127]
		Randomized, double-blind, placebo controlled trial in healthy overweight older adults for 26 weeks	Resveratrol 200 mg/d (23 subjects) *vs* placebo (23 subjects)	Resveratrol group showed a significant reduction in HbA1c and body fat compared with placebo.	[128]

(Table 1) cont.....

Name of the Possible Phytoremedies Studied	Plant Part/ Phytoconstituents/ Materials used/composition	Study Design & Duration	Dosage and Groups	Outcomes	References
Scoparia dulcis	Porridge was packed (40 g) in air tight packets which contained fresh leaves: rice: scraped coconut kernel in 13–15: 25–30: 10–13 (w/w/w) ratios (Phytoconstituents: Diterpenes, triterpenes, flavonoids)	Randomized crossover clinical trial for 3 months	Cross-over clinical trials in which diabetes test group (35 patients) consumed commercially produced SDC for 3 days/week for 3 months and control group received other food	Porridge reduced HbA1c level, non-significant reduction in FBG, plasma insulin, and cholesterol levels.	[129]
Semen Persical decoction for purgation with addition (SPDPA)- TCM Formulation	SPDPA formula: Rhubarb 6~12 g, Semen Persical 9-12 g, Ramulus Cinnamomum 6~12 g; dried Glauber's salt 3~6g, Radix Glycyrrhizae 3~6 g, Radix Scrophularie 12~15 g, Radix Rehmanniae dried or prepared 12~15 g, Radix Ophiopogonis 12 g and Radix Astragalus 30-~45 g	Non-randomized, open-label, 2 parallel groups for 2 months	T2DM patients (148) received a dose of SPDPA daily Control group: Received glyburide only.	Decreased FBG; the changes of FBG was similar with glibenclamide. No side-effect	[130]
Soy bean *(Glycine max)*	Pinitol with 95% purity was prepared from soybean by water extraction	Randomized, double-blind, placebo controlled trial in T2DM patients for 13 weeks	T2DM patients (30), Pinitol dose:1200 mg/d (15 patients) *vs.* placebo (15 patients)	Pinitol significantly decreased mean fasting plasma glucose, insulin, fructosamine, HbA1c, and the homeostatic model assessment insulin resistance index.	[131]
Stevia rebaudiana	Steviol glycoside capsules 250 mg	Randomized, double-blind, placebo controlled, parallel, study in T2DM patients for 3 months	76 subjects (30 with Type 2 diabetes, 16 with Type 1 diabetes and 30 without diabetes The subjects in each group were randomly allocated to active treatment (the steviol glycoside 250 mg t.d.s.) or to placebo treatment.	Post-treatment systolic BP, diastolic BP, glucose and glycated hemoglobin (HbA1c) were not significantly different from baseline measurements, except for the placebo Type 1 diabetics group where a significant difference was observed for systolic BP and glucose. No side-effects were observed in the two treatment groups.	[132]
Tibetan Medicine herb combination	Tibetan medicine herbs: individualized powder/pill combination	Open-label, 2 parallel groups newly diagnosed or untreated patients on diet alone for 6 months	T2DM patients (200) received Tibetan medicine herbs: Individualized powder/pill combination (at least 2 of 4: Kyura-6, Aru-18, Yungwa-4, Sugmel-19) Control: No herb treatment	Decreased FPG, PPG, and glycated hemoglobin (GHb); no observed change in weight.	[134]

(Table 1) cont.....

Name of the Possible Phytoremedies Studied	Plant Part/ Phytoconstituents/ Materials used/composition	Study Design & Duration	Dosage and Groups	Outcomes	References
Traditional Chinese Treatment (TCT)	Combination of *Coptis chinensis, Astragalus membranaceus* and *Lonicera japonica*	Double-blind, 4 parallel groups study on diet alone for for 3 months	T2DM patients (216), TCT herb: 21 capsules/d (each containing 150 mg *Coptis chinensis*, 30 mg *Astragalus membranaceus*, 120 mg *Lonicera japonica*) along with Oral Hypoglycemic agent (glibenclamide 7.5 mg/d) Control: Placebo TCT capsule or placebo OHA tablet	Decreased FBG and PPG with synergistic effect of both treatments. No change in insulin or HgbA1C.	[135]
Tulsi/Holy basil *(Ocimum sanctum)*	Leaves powder (Phytoconstituents: Caryophylline protein-bound polysaccharide carvacrol, linalool)	Single-blind, crossover, patients on diet and/or OHA for 4 weeks	T2DM patients (40), fresh leaves powder: 2.5 g Control: Fresh spinach leaves powder	Decreased FBG, PPG and urine glucose. No side-effect was observed.	[136]
Ulam raja *(Cosmos caudatus)*	Vacuum packed fresh leaves (contains ascorbic acid, quercetin, proanthocyanidin, chlorogenic acid and catechin phytocompounds)	Single center, randomized, controlled, two-arms parallel design clinical trial for 8 weeks	diabetic-ulam group (38) consumed 15 g of *C. caudatus* daily while diabetic control group (39) abstained from taking *C. caudatus*	*C. caudatus* significantly reduced serum insulin, homeostatic model assessment-insulin resistance and increased quantitative insulin sensitivity check index in diabetic-ulam group compared with the diabetic controls. HbA1C level was improved although it is not statistically significant	[137]
Vanadium	Vanadyl sulfate hydrate	Non-randomized, single-blind, crossover study with diet and/or OHA for 3 weeks	Type 2 diabetic patients (6) received vanadyl sulfate hydrate: 100 mg/day Control: Placebo capsule	Decreased FBG, HbA1c, hepatic glucose production, increased insulin-mediated glucose uptake, insulin sensitivity. No changed in PPG and C-peptide levels.	[138]
	Vanadyl sulfate hydrate	Non-randomized, single-blind crossover study for 3 weeks	Type 2 diabetic patients (7) received vanadyl sulfate hydrate: 100 mg/day Control: Placebo capsule	Decreased FBG, HbA1c, hepatic glucose output and increased insulin sensitivity but no change in insulin level.	[139]
	Vanadyl sulfate	Non-randomized, single-blind, crossover study with OHA and/or insulin for 4 weeks	Type 2 diabetic patients (8) received vanadyl sulfate: 100 mg/d Control: Placebo capsule	Decreased FBG, hepatic glucose output during clamp.	[140]
	Vanadyl sulfate	Noncontrolled open-label studies for 6 weeks	Type 2 diabetic patients (11) received vanadyl sulfate: 150 mg/day	Improved hepatic and muscle insulin sensitivity in T2DM diabetic patients.	[141]
	Sodium metavanadate	Noncontrolled open-label studies for 2 weeks	5 IDDM and 5 NIDDM patients received oral sodium metavanadate: 125 mg/day	Significant decrease in insulin requirements in patients with IDDM. Cholesterol levels significantly decreased in both IDDM and NIDDM.	[142]

(Table 1) cont.....

Name of the Possible Phytoremedies Studied	Plant Part/ Phytoconstituents/ Materials used/composition	Study Design & Duration	Dosage and Groups	Outcomes	References
Vit C	Sodium ascorbate		10 diabetic subjects and 10 nondiabetic control subjects; diabetic subjects received treatment with diet alone (n = 2), diet plus oral sulfonylurea (n = 6), or diet plus insulin injections (24 mg/min) (n = 2).	Infusion of vitamin C stimulated the vasodilating activity of methacholine, whereas vasodilation to nitroprusside and to verapamil remained unaffected by vitamin C. On the other hand, endothelium-dependent vasodilation was not affected by vitamin C infusion.	[150]
			10 healthy subjects and 10 type II diabetic patients; vitamin C infusion rate (0.9 mmol/min)	Vitamin C infusion increased insulin action	[151]
Vit E		Double-blind; Crossover, well controlled on diet and OHA for 4 months	15 Type 2 diabetic patients; Vitamin E; 900 mg/d dlalpha-tocopheryl acetate Control: Sodium citrate placebo	Decreased HbA1c, FPG and PPG. No change in insulin, hepatic glucose output and glucose oxidation. Increased total body glucose disposal and non-oxidative glucose metabolism.	[152]
		Double-blind, 2 parallel groups on diet and/or OHA received Vit-E for 10 weeks	Type 2 diabetes patients (21) received Vitamin E: 1600 IU/d d-alpha tocopherol Control: Placebo pill	No change in FBG, PPG, postprandial insulin, glycated Hgb, glycated albumin, glycated total plasma proteins, fructosamine; decreased susceptibility of LDL to oxidation No side effects	[153]
		Single-blind, 3 parallel groups, on diet and insulin for 2 months	Insulin-requiring diabetes mellitus patients (30) received Vitamin E: 1200 mg/d *vs* 600 mg/d (unspecified preparation). Control: Placebo	Decreased HbA1c and glycosylated protein (dose related), No change in FPG or mean daily glucose.	[154]
		Double-blind, crossover, well controlled on diet and OHA for 3 months	Type 2 diabetic patients (25) received Vitamin E: 900 mg/d d-alphatocopherol Control: Placebo pill	Decreased FPG, HbA1c, and PPG. No change in insulin.	[155]
		Double-blind; crossover, poorly controlled on diet, OHA and/or insulin for 2 months	53 T2DM diabetic patients (39 Type 2, 14 Type 1) received Vitamin E: 1200 mg/d Control: Placebo capsule	No change in FBG, Fructosamine and HbA1c.	[156]
		Non-randomized, double-blind, 2 parallel groups for 3 months	Type 1 diabetic patients (35) received Vitamin E: 100 IU/d. Control: Placebo capsule	Decreased HbA1c but no changed in FPG and insulin requirement.	[157]

(Table 1) cont.....

Name of the Possible Phytoremedies Studied	Plant Part/ Phytoconstituents/ Materials used/composition	Study Design & Duration	Dosage and Groups	Outcomes	References
Walnut oil (*Juglan sregia* L.)	Persian walnut was cold pressed to extract the oil from them	Randomized, double-blind, placebo-controlled clinical trial 90 days	Hyperlipidemic T2DM patients (100), 4 walnut oil capsules containing 1.25 cc walnut oil, three times daily with food (15 cc daily); 4 placebo capsules containing 1.25 cc distilled water, three times daily with food (15 cc daily)	Addition of walnut oil in the daily diet of type 2 diabetic patients improves lipid profile	[158]
White mulberry (*Morus alba*)	Ethanol extract of white murlberry leaves (phytoconstituent: 1-Deoxynojirimycin)	Randomized, double-blind, placebo controlled trial in subjects with impaired glucose metabolism for 3 months	1-deoxynojirimycin: 18 mg/d before meal (33 patients) *vs.* placebo (32 patients)	Improved postprandial glycemic control in individuals with impaired glucose metabolism.	[159]
Xiaoke pill –TCM Preparation	The herb components include Radix Puerariae, Radix Rehmanniae, Radix Astragali, Radix Trichosanthis, Stylus Zeae Maydis, Fructus Schisandrae Sphenantherae, and Rhizoma Dioscoreae with 0.25 microgram of glibenclamide per pill	Controlled, double blind, multicentre non-inferiority trial for 48 weeks	800 patients (drug naive group, n= 400) or add on therapy (metformin group, n = 400) with Xiaoke pill or Glibenclamide tablet	Xiaoke Pill significantly reduced the total hypoglycemia rate and the mild hypoglycemic episode and improved blood glucose levels in both groups compared to glibenclamide during the follow-up period of 48 weeks	[160]

*All trials are randomized unless otherwise specified.

White Mulberry *(Morus alba)*

Morus alba (known as mulberry) leaves conatin 1-deoxynojirimycin (DNJ) which possesses significant inhibitory action to α-glucosidase. Asai *et al.* performed two randomized, double-blind, crossover trials on individuals with dysfunction in glucose metabolism. 12 individuals were tested using either single ingestion of mulberry leaf extract (3, 6 or 9 mg DNJ) or placebo after 2 hours of carbohydrate intake (200 g boiled white rice) in the first trial and in the second trial, 76 individuals were allocated to receive mulberry extract (6 mg DNJ, thrice daily) for 12 weeks. The findings of both trials indicated improvement in postprandial glucose levels of individuals with impaired glucose metabolism after supplementing with mulberry leaf extract [159].

Xiaoke Pill (TCM Preparation)

In 2013, a double blind, multicentre non-inferiority trial enrolled 800 type 2 diabetic patients with poorly controlled blood glucose level and randomly divided them into two groups: drug naive group and metformin group (patients previously taken metformin monotherapy). The patients were administered either Xiaoke Pill (a compound of Chinese herbs combined with glibenclamide), or Glibenclamide for 4 weeks. The trial showed that Xiaoke Pill significantly reduced the total hypoglycemia rate and the mild hypoglycemic episode and improved blood glucose levels in both groups compared to glibenclamide during the follow-up period of 48 weeks [160].

DISCUSSION

This chapter presents the updated panorama of phytomedicines (herbal preparations, plant extracts, bioactive phyto-compounds, traditional herbal medicines, functional foods, nutraceuticals, vitamins and mineral supplements) with the evidences of clinical studies/trials for the management of diabetes mellitus. The considered outcomes for the clinical effectiveness of phytoremedies against the diabetes were significant reduction of fasting blood glucose, post-prandial blood glucose, HbA1c levels as well as significant improvement in insulin sensitivity, HOMA-IR, glucose uptake and storage, lipid profile and blood pressure of the patients. The occurrence of adverse-effects and other aspects of safety profile were also considered for the evaluation of therapeutic value of those phytotherapies.

Based on the outcomes of the clinical studies of phytomedicine candidates presented here, several of them demonstrated to be very effective with good safety profile, even better than that of the respective Allopathic antidiabetic drugs currently available for the treatment of diabetes. For example, berberine-the bioactive compound obtained from *Berberis aristata*, demonstrated similar effectiveness with metformin as monotherapy in newly diagnosed T2DM patients to improve the level of HbA1c, FPG, PPBG, basal insulin and postprandial insulin levels. This indicates the similar effectiveness of berberine and metformin in the management of glucose metabolism and insulin secretion [37]. Berberine was also reported to significantly improve the levels of HbA1c, FPG, PBG, basal insulin, HOMA-IR, fasting and postprandial C-peptide as adjuvant therapy in poorly controlled T2DM patients [37]. Besides, several other studies confirmed the antidiabetic effectiveness of berberine as strong as metformin or rosiglitazone to control the hepatic glucose and improvement of insulin sensitivity. The additional advantage of berberine over metformin and rosiglitazone is that berberine is effective to manage glycemic profile in patients with hepatitis, thus it can be as a replacement or adjuvant therapy with conventional antidiabetic agents that cannot be used in case of hepatitis. For example, metformin and rosiglitazone have been shown to exhibit hepatic side-effects [39]. Moreover, berberine was reported to exhibit antihyperlipidemic and anti-inflammatory activities which may contribute additional benefits in the management of diabetes mellitus [42, 43]. Thus, berberine could be a better choice for the management of diabetes comparing to the currently available respective antidiabetic medicaments, especially for the treatment of patients with hepatitis or to avoid the adverse effects of liver.

Another potential antidiabetic phytotherapy is Bitter gourd *(Momordica charantia),* which is eaten as vegetables all over the world. Because of the presence of charantin, vicine, and polypeptide-p (an unidentified insulin-like protein) phytoconstituents, it works as an excellent functional food to improve glycemic control [48]. Many clinical studies reported the potentiality of fruit juice, extract, powder, and its isolated bioactive compounds to reduce fasting, post-prandial, random blood glucose levels, HbA1c, bad cholesterols, insulin levels, glucose uptake and utilization. As bitter gourd is a functional food, its safety profile is very high; thus can be used as antidiabetic phytotherapy avoiding the adverse-effects usually occur in the case of conventional drugs [49 - 52].

Cinnamon (*Cinnamomum zeylanicum*), likewise bitter gourd, is another functional food that is used as a popular cooking spice. Because of the presence of cinnamaldehyde and some other flavonoid compounds, it has fantastic glucose lowering ability resulted from the clinical trials of many studies. Systematic review of clinical studies demonstrated that cinnamon powder and extracts have the potential ability to control elevated blood glucose, reducing TG and LDL-c, and increasing HDL-c levels in diabetes patients. No adverse effects were reported with the used therapeutic doses [67].

Fenugreek and Nigella are two functional foods that resulted with potential effects to control fasting, post-prandial blood glucose levels and HbA1c as well as to stimulate the sensitivity of resistant insulin. Sharma *et al.* reported that fenugreek improved glycemic control in case of not only type 2 diabetes mellitus but also type 1 diabetes mellitus as well [78]. Meta-analysis of clinical trials of *Nigella sativa* resulted in significant control of hyperglycemia, lipid profile of diabetes patients [111]. The mechanism behind the glucose lowering capability of fenugreek is to stimulate the sensitivity of resistant insulin and improvement of glucose uptake and utilization. Whereas, *Nigella sativa* exerts its antidiabetic capability by amelioration of pancreatic β-cells leading to insulin secretion, reducing hepatic gluconeogenesis, and inducing insulin sensitivity in peripheral tissue due to its active phytocompounds thymoquinone, dithymoquinone, linoleic acid and oleic acid [112 - 118].

Several other phytomaterials have been shown to have prospective results as potential antidiabetic phytoremedies for the treatment of diabetes, avoiding side-effects and contraindication of conventional drugs. For example, Yongchaiyudha, *et al.* reported that aloe gel has potential in treating diabetes because it can lower not only sugar but also triglyceride levels, which are often high in diabetic patients. The study also showed that aloe gel had no adverse-effect on kidney and liver functions [32]. Na *et al.*, showed that supplementation with curcuminoids over a three-month period at a dose of 300 mg/day results in a significant improvement in glycemic control in type 2 diabetic patients. This might be due to a decrease in serum fatty acid, possibly through the promotion of fatty acid oxidation and utilization [51]. Vuksan *et al.* suggested that American ginseng might be important for individuals with type 2 diabetes mellitus to take ginseng with meals [55]. Therefore, ginseng may be a useful therapeutic adjunct in the management of NIDDM. Resveratrol supplementation could also be used as an effective adjuvant therapy with a conventional hypoglycemic regimen to treat T2DM since it improves glycemic control and the associated risk factors in patients with T2DM [57]. Gymnema increases the enzyme activity responsible for glucose uptake and utilization as well as stimulates β-cell function, increases β-cell number, and/or increases insulin release by increasing cell permeability to insulin. No side-effects have been reported secondary to gymnema use [30].

Some commercially available herbal preparations have reported very prospective results in the treatment of diabetes resulted from the clinical trials. For example, Dia-Best™ is a commercially available polyherbal dietary supplement, as mentioned previously. Oral administration of 3g powder of Dia-Best™ in a sachet in the morning 20 minutes before breakfast and at night 1 hour before sleep for 2 months in clinical study with type 2 diabetes patients resulted with potential improvement of fasting blood glucose levels (11.63 mmoL/L to 8.92 mmoL/L), post-prandial blood glucose levels (19.66 to 13.82 mmoL/L), HbA1c (8.9% to 7.2%), total serum cholesterol (p<0.01), LDL-c (p<0.01), and TG (p<0.001). No adverse effects were observed in any patient. Rather, some diabetes patients reported better and comfortable fecal clearance who had constipation or irregular defaecation [76]]. Another commercial phytotherapeutic preparation is GlucoSupreme™ Herbal. In a multi-site, double-blinded, randomized controlled clinical trial with prediabetes for 12 weeks resulted in restoring glycemic parameters to normal ranges, irrespective of broad changes in diet or physical activity. Thus, this product can be used for the prevention of T2DM [89].

A randomized, double-blind, placebo-controlled clinical studies with *Stevia rebaudiana* and its isolated active ingredient (steviol glycosides) with diabetes patients resulted no improvement of serum glucose, HbA1c, and blood pressure compared to placebo. It is noteworthy to mention here that many diabetes patients traditionally use stevia for the treatment of diabetes from their belief that it has antidiabetic activity. Analysing the clinical study results, it can be concluded that stevia is not effective and cannot be recommended as an antidiabetic phytoremedy, rather stevia can be used as an alternative to sugar for the preparation of antidiabetic phytomedicines and for the consumption of diabetes patients [132].

Micronutrients such as chromium, magnesium, vanadium, vitamin C, and vitamin E were reported to possess antidiabetic activities through different mechanisms. Hypomagnesemia causes insulin resistance, observed in diabetes patients. Magnesium has been reported to improve insulin sensitivity, post-prandial insulin secretion, FBG and HbA1c [101 - 103] in diabetes. Few small scale clinical studies reported antidiabetic activities of palladium but its use as antidiabetic therapy cannot be recommended without sufficient evidences. Although several clinical studies were performed on chromium, some studies reported its antidiabetic ability but some reported no change in the glucose levels, insulin sensitivity, and other diabetes-related parameters.

Phytopreparations, such as, *Artocarpus heterophyllus,* Carnitine, *Apium graveolens,* Corn Bran, *Ficus carica, Mellissa officinalis* based product, Onion (*Allium cepa*), *Opuntia streptacantha, Scoparia dulcis, Soybean,* Holy basil (*Ocimum sanctum*) and Walnut oil *(Juglan sregia)* provided insufficient evidence or different/inconsistent outcomes which made difficult to recommend them as antidiabetic phytomedicines.

Evidences from both the experimental and clinical studies suggest that oxidative stress plays a major role in the pathogenesis of both types of diabetes mellitus. In diabetes, free radicals are formed disproportionately by oxidation of glucose, nonenzymatic glycation of proteins, and the oxidative degradation of glycated proteins [161]. Abnormally high levels of free radicals and the simultaneous decline of antioxidant defence mechanisms can lead to damage of cellular organelles and enzymes, increased lipid peroxidation, and development of insulin resistance [161]. Increasing lipid peroxidation has a close relationship with high glucose levels in diabetes mellitus, which can be observed in FBG and HbA1c levels. Oxidative stress acts as a mediator of insulin resistance, progression to glucose intolerance, installation of DM, consequently favours the generation of atherosclerotic complications [162]. In case of severe oxidative stress, pancreatic beta cells become sensitive to reactive oxygen and nitrogen species due to the low expression of antioxidant enzymes [163]. These molecules may act on different substrates in the insulin intracellular signaling cascade, ultimately resulting in pancreatic cell damage [164]. Mechanisms by which increased oxidative stress is involved in the diabetic complications are partly known, including activation of transcription factors, advanced glycated end products (AGEs), and protein kinase C [161]. These consequences of oxidative stress can promote the development of complications of diabetes mellitus.

Antioxidants are very important for the prevention of diabetes and protection of pancreatic beta-cells damage. Vitamin C is an important antioxidant that has strong ability for the scavenging of oxygen-derived free radicals. Studies found that the levels of vitamin C in diabetic patients is 40-50% lower than its normal level found in nondiabetic subjects [144 - 149]. Vitamin C promotes insulin action, mainly with the enhancement of non-oxidative glucose metabolism [151].

CONCLUDING REMARKS

Multiple clinical study results demonstrated very prospective and potential antidiabetic activities of the following phytoremedies: Berberine, Bitter gourd, Cinnamon, Curcumin, Dia-Best™, Fenugreek, Gegen Qinlian decoction, GlucoSupreme herbal, *Gymnema sylvestre*, Magnesium, *Nigella sativa*, Resveratrol, Tibetan medicine herb combination, TCM multiple herbal combination, Xiaoke pill, and vitamin C. Therefore, these phytoremedies are strongly recommended for the management of type 2 diabetes mellitus. Based on the results from clinical studies, we can conclude that Aloe vera, α-lipoic acid, Chromium, *Coccinia indica*, Chamomile, Ginseng, Green tea, Milk thistle, SPDPA, *Pinus pinaster, Scoparia dulcis,* Soybean, Ulam Raja and White Marlberry phytoremedies may be useful for the management of type 2 diabetes mellitus. Because of the lack of sufficient evidences or inconsistent outcomes or no positive changes for its antidiabetic activities, *Artocarpus heterophyllus,* Bell pepper, Carnitine, *Apium graveolens,* Corn bran, *Ficus carica, Mellissa officinalis* based product, *Humulus lupulus,* Onion, *Opuntia streptacantha,* Red clover, *Scoparia dulcis*, Soybean, Holy basil, Lignan from Flaxseed, *Myrcia uniflora,* Vanadium, Vitamin E, and Wall nut oil are not recommended to use for the management of type 2 diabetes mellitus. The clinical study reports presented here can be very useful to provide important information and source of knowledge for the students, academicians, researchers, industry people, alternative medicine practitioners to use the prospective and therapeutically important phytomedicines as the elements for the preparation of alternative medicines or for direct use as an alternative medicine or for further research for the discovery and development of new Allopathic medicine/pharmaceutical products for the effective treatment of type 2 diabetes mellitus by minimizing or avoiding the side-effects and limitations of conventional medicines.

CONSENT FOR PUBLICATION

Not applicable.

CONFLICT OF INTEREST

There is no conflict of interest declared.

ACKNOWLEDGEMENT

The authors would like to acknowledge the Department of Pharmacy, State University of Bangladesh, and Health Med Science Research Limited to provide facilities to produce the book chapter.

LIST OF ABBREVIATIONS

T2DM	type 2 diabetes mellitus
NIDDM	Non-insulin dependent diabetes mellitus
GDM	Gestational diabetes mellitus
FBG	Fasting blood glucose
PPBG	Post-prandial blood glucose
PBG	Plasma blood glucose
HbA1c	Glycated hemoglobin or Hemoglobin A1c
OGTT	Oral glucose tolerance test
OHA	Oral hypoglycemic agent
LDL-c	low density lipoprotein-c
HDL-c	High density lipoprotein-c
HOMA-IR	Homeostatic Model Assessment of Insulin Resistance
ND	not determined
LSI	Life-style intervention
TCM	Traditional Chinese medicine
SGOT	serum glutamic-oxaloacetic transaminase
SGPT	Serum glutamic pyruvic transaminase
TAG	triacylglycerol
SBP	Systolic blood pressure
BBR	Berberine
PGZ	Pioglitazone
CHB	Corn Bran Hemicellulose
FSIVGTT	Frequently sampled intravenous glucose tolerance test
SGLT2	Sodium glucose co-transporter-2 inhibitors
DPP-4	Dipeptidyl peptidase - 4 inhibitors
GLP	Glucagon-like peptide-1
GIP	Gastric inhibitory polypeptide
AGEs	Advanced glycated end products.

REFERENCES

[1]   World Health Organization. Classification of Diabetes Mellitus. 2019. Available online: https://apps.who.int/iris/bitstream/handle/10665/325182/9789241515702-eng.pdf?sequence=1& isAllowed=y

[2]   American Diabetes Association. Classification and diagnosis of diabetes: standards of medical care in diabetes - 2019. Diabetes Care 2018; 41 (Suppl. 1): S13-27.
[http://dx.doi.org/10.2337/dc18-S002] [PMID: 29222373]

[3]   Report of a World Health Organization consultation. Use of glycated haemoglobin (HbA1c) in the diagnosis of diabetes mellitus. Diabetes Res Clin Pract 2011; 93: 299-309.
[http://dx.doi.org/10.1016/j.diabres.2011.03.012]

[4]   World Health Organization. Diabetes: Key Facts. 2018. Available online: https://www.who.int/ news-room/ fact-sheets/detail/diabetes

[5]   International Diabetes Federation. About diabetes: Diabetes facts & figures. 2017. Available online: https://www.who.int/news-room/ fact-sheets/detail/ diabetes

[6]   Nickerson HD, Dutta S. Diabetic complications: current challenges and opportunities. J Cardiovasc Transl Res 2012; 5(4): 375-9.
[http://dx.doi.org/10.1007/s12265-012-9388-1] [PMID: 22752737]

[7]   Giovannucci E, Harlan DM, Archer MC, *et al.* Diabetes and cancer: a consensus report. CA Cancer J Clin 2010; 60(4): 207-21.
[http://dx.doi.org/10.3322/caac.20078] [PMID: 20554718]

[8]   Song R. Mechanism of Metformin: A Tale of Two Sites. Diabetes Care 2016; 39(2): 187-9.
[http://dx.doi.org/10.2337/dci15-0013] [PMID: 26798149]

[9]   Ganesan K, Sultan S. Oral Hypoglycemic Medications. StatPearls. StatPearls Publishing 2019.

[10]   https://www.accessdata.fda.gov/drugsatfda_docs/label/2006/021748s002lbl.pdf

[11]   Marín-Peñalver JJ, Martín-Timón I, Sevillano-Collantes C, Del Cañizo-Gómez FJ. Update on the treatment of type 2 diabetes mellitus. World J Diabetes 2016; 7(17): 354-95.
[http://dx.doi.org/10.4239/wjd.v7.i17.354] [PMID: 27660695]

[12]   Guardado-Mendoza R, Prioletta A, Jiménez-Ceja LM, Sosale A, Folli F. The role of nateglinide and repaglinide, derivatives of meglitinide, in the treatment of type 2 diabetes mellitus. Arch Med Sci 2013; 9(5): 936-43.
[http://dx.doi.org/10.5114/aoms.2013.34991] [PMID: 24273582]

[13]   Taheri Rouhi SZ, Sarker MMR, Rahmat A, Alkahtani SA, Othman F. The effect of pomegranate fresh juice *versus* pomegranate seed powder on metabolic indices, lipid profile, inflammatory biomarkers, and the histopathology of pancreatic islets of Langerhans in streptozotocin-nicotinamide induced type 2 diabetic Sprague-Dawley rats. BMC Complement Altern Med 2017; 17(1): 156.
[http://dx.doi.org/10.1186/s12906-017-1667-6] [PMID: 28288617]

[14]   Shah MA, Sarker MMR, Gousuddin M. Antidiabetic potential of *Brassica Oleracea* Var. Italica in type 2 diabetic sprague dawley (sd) rats. Int J Pharmacogn Phytochem Res 2016; 8(3): 462-9.

[15]   Sarker MMR, Zihad MATR, Islam M, *et al.* Antihyperglycemic, insulin-sensitivity and anti-hyperlipidemic potential of *Ganoderma lucidum*, a dietary mushroom, on alloxan- and glucocorticoid-induced diabetic Long-Evans rats. Funct Food Health Dis 2015; 5(12): 450-66.
[http://dx.doi.org/10.31989/ffhd.v5i12.220]

[16]   Chen Y, Liu Y, Sarker MMR, *et al.* Structural characterization and antidiabetic potential of a novel heteropolysaccharide from *Grifola frondosa via* IRS1/PI3K-JNK signaling pathways. Carbohydr Polym 2018; 198: 452-61.
[http://dx.doi.org/10.1016/j.carbpol.2018.06.077] [PMID: 30093022]

[17]　Sheikh BY, Sarker MMR, Kamarudin MNA, Ismail A. Prophetic medicine as potential functional food elements in the intervention of cancer: A review. Biomed Pharmacother 2017; 95: 614-48. a [http://dx.doi.org/10.1016/j.biopha.2017.08.043] [PMID: 28888208]

[18]　Sheikh BY, Sarker MMR, Kamarudin MNA, Mohan G. Antiproliferative and apoptosis inducing effects of citral *via* p53 and ROS-induced mitochondrial-mediated apoptosis in human colorectal HCT116 and HT29 cell lines. Biomed Pharmacother 2017; 96: 834-46. b [http://dx.doi.org/10.1016/j.biopha.2017.10.038] [PMID: 29078261]

[19]　Goto T, Sarker MMR, Zhong M, Tanaka S, Gohda E. Enhancement of immunoglobulin M production in B cells by the extract of red bell pepper. J Health Sci 2010; 56(3): 304-9. [http://dx.doi.org/10.1248/jhs.56.304]

[20]　Sarker MMR, Gohda E. Promotion of anti-keyhole limpet hemocyanin IgM and IgG antibody productions *in vitro* by red bell pepper extract. J Funct Foods 2013; 5(4): 1918-26. [http://dx.doi.org/10.1016/j.jff.2013.09.013]

[21]　Sarker MMR, Nahar S, Shahriar M, Seraj S, Choudhuri MSK. Preliminary study of the immunostimulating activity of an ayurvedic preparation, Kanakasava, on the splenic cells of BALB/c mice *in vitro*. Pharm Biol 2012; 50(11): 1467-72. a [http://dx.doi.org/10.3109/13880209.2012.681329] [PMID: 22849578]

[22]　Sarker MMR, Nimmi I, Kawsar MH. Preliminary screening of six popular fruits of Bangladesh for *in vitro* IgM production and proliferation of splenocytes. Bangladesh Pharm J 2012; 15(1): 31-7. b

[23]　Sarker MMR, Mazumder MEH, Rashid MHO. *In vitro* enhancement of polyclonal IgM production by ethanolic extract of *Nigella sativa* L. seeds in whole spleen cells of female BALB/c mice. Bangladesh Pharm J 2011; 14(1): 73-7.

[24]　Kazemipoor M, Cordell GA, Sarker MMR, Radzi CWJBWM, Hajifaraji M. En Kiat P. Alternative treatments for weight loss: Safety/risks and effectiveness of anti-obesity medicinal plants. Int J Food Prop 2015; 18(9): 1942-63. [http://dx.doi.org/10.1080/10942912.2014.933350]

[25]　Imam H, Mahbub NU, Khan MF, Hana HK, Sarker MMR. Alpha amylase enzyme inhibitory and anti-inflammatory effect of Lawsonia inermis. Pak J Biol Sci 2013; 16(23): 1796-800. [http://dx.doi.org/10.3923/pjbs.2013.1796.1800] [PMID: 24506051]

[26]　Yasmin H, Kaiser MA, Sarker MMR, Rahman MS, Rashid MA. Preliminary anti-bacterial activity of some indigenous plants of Bangladesh. Dhaka Univ J Pharm Sci 2009; 8(1): 61-5. [http://dx.doi.org/10.3329/dujps.v8i1.5337]

[27]　Pandey VN, Rajagopalan SS, Chowdhary DP. An effective Ayurvedic hypoglycemic formulation. J Res Ayurveda Siddha 1995; 16(1-2): 1-4.

[28]　Shane-McWhorter L. Biological complementary therapies: a focus on botanical products in diabetes. Diabetes Spectr 2001; 14(4): 199-208. [http://dx.doi.org/10.2337/diaspect.14.4.199]

[29]　Bunyapraphatsara N, Yongchaiyudha S, Rungpitarangsi V, Chokechaijaroenporn O. Antidiabetic activity of *Aloe vera* L. juice II. Clinical trial in diabetes mellitus patients in combination with glibenclamide. Phytomedicine 1996; 3(3): 245-8. [http://dx.doi.org/10.1016/S0944-7113(96)80061-4] [PMID: 23195078]

[30]　Yongchaiyudha S, Rungpitarangsi V, Bunyapraphatsara N, Chokechaijaroenporn O. Antidiabetic activity of *Aloe vera* L. juice. I. Clinical trial in new cases of diabetes mellitus. Phytomedicine 1996; 3(3): 241-3. [http://dx.doi.org/10.1016/S0944-7113(96)80060-2] [PMID: 23195077]

[31]　Ghannam N, Kingston M, Al-Meshaal IA, Tariq M, Parman NS, Woodhouse N. The antidiabetic activity of aloes: preliminary clinical and experimental observations. Horm Res 1986; 24(4): 288-94. [http://dx.doi.org/10.1159/000180569] [PMID: 3096865]

[32] Huseini HF, Kianbakht S, Hajiaghaee R, Dabaghian FH. Anti-hyperglycemic and anti-hypercholesterolemic effects of Aloe vera leaf gel in hyperlipidemic type 2 diabetic patients: a randomized double-blind placebo-controlled clinical trial. Planta Med 2012; 78(4): 311-6.
[http://dx.doi.org/10.1055/s-0031-1280474] [PMID: 22198821]

[33] Jacob S, Ruus P, Hermann R, *et al.* Oral administration of RAC-α-lipoic acid modulates insulin sensitivity in patients with type-2 diabetes mellitus: a placebo-controlled pilot trial. Free Radic Biol Med 1999; 27(3-4): 309-14.
[http://dx.doi.org/10.1016/S0891-5849(99)00089-1] [PMID: 10468203]

[34] Konrad T, Vicini P, Kusterer K, *et al.* alpha-Lipoic acid treatment decreases serum lactate and pyruvate concentrations and improves glucose effectiveness in lean and obese patients with type 2 diabetes. Diabetes Care 1999; 22(2): 280-7.
[http://dx.doi.org/10.2337/diacare.22.2.280] [PMID: 10333946]

[35] Fernando MR, Wickramasinghe N, Thabrew MI, Ariyananda PL, Karunanayake EH. Effect of *Artocarpus heterophyllus* and *Asteracanthus longifolia* on glucose tolerance in normal human subjects and in maturity-onset diabetic patients. J Ethnopharmacol 1991; 31(3): 277-82.
[http://dx.doi.org/10.1016/0378-8741(91)90012-3] [PMID: 2056756]

[36] Nagasukeerthi P, Mooventhan A, Manjunath NK. Short-term effect of add on bell pepper (*Capsicum annuum* var. grossum) juice with integrated approach of yoga therapy on blood glucose levels and cardiovascular functions in patients with type 2 diabetes mellitus: A randomized controlled study. Complement Ther Med 2017; 34: 42-5.
[http://dx.doi.org/10.1016/j.ctim.2017.07.011] [PMID: 28917374]

[37] Yin J, Xing H, Ye J. Efficacy of berberine in patients with type 2 diabetes mellitus. Metabolism 2008; 57(5): 712-7.
[http://dx.doi.org/10.1016/j.metabol.2008.01.013] [PMID: 18442638]

[38] Zhang Y, Li X, Zou D, *et al.* Treatment of type 2 diabetes and dyslipidemia with the natural plant alkaloid berberine. J Clin Endocrinol Metab 2008; 93(7): 2559-65.
[http://dx.doi.org/10.1210/jc.2007-2404] [PMID: 18397984]

[39] Zhang H, Wei J, Xue R, *et al.* Berberine lowers blood glucose in type 2 diabetes mellitus patients through increasing insulin receptor expression. Metabolism 2010; 59(2): 285-92.
[http://dx.doi.org/10.1016/j.metabol.2009.07.029] [PMID: 19800084]

[40] Gu Y, Zhang Y, Shi X, *et al.* Effect of traditional Chinese medicine berberine on type 2 diabetes based on comprehensive metabonomics. Talanta 2010; 81(3): 766-72.
[http://dx.doi.org/10.1016/j.talanta.2010.01.015] [PMID: 20298851]

[41] Yan HM, Xia MF, Wang Y, *et al.* Efficacy of berberine in patients with non-alcoholic fatty liver disease. PLoS One 2015; 10(8)e0134172
[http://dx.doi.org/10.1371/journal.pone.0134172] [PMID: 26252777]

[42] Chen L, Lu W, Li Y. Berberine ameliorates type 2 diabetes *via* modulation of Bifidobacterium species, tumor necrosis factor-alpha, and lipopolysaccharide. Int J Clin Exp Med 2016; 9(6): 9365-72.

[43] Lazavi F, Mirmiran P, Sohrab G, Nikpayam O, Angoorani P, Hedayati M. The barberry juice effects on metabolic factors and oxidative stress in patients with type 2 diabetes: A randomized clinical trial. Complement Ther Clin Pract 2018; 31: 170-4.
[http://dx.doi.org/10.1016/j.ctcp.2018.01.009] [PMID: 29705451]

[44] Derosa G, D'Angelo A, Romano D, Maffioli P. Effects of a combination of *Berberis aristata, Silybum marianum* and monacolin on lipid profile in subjects at low cardiovascular risk; a double-blind, randomized, placebo-controlled trial. Int J Mol Sci 2017; 18(2): 343.
[http://dx.doi.org/10.3390/ijms18020343] [PMID: 28178209]

[45] Di Pierro F, Villanova N, Agostini F, Marzocchi R, Soverini V, Marchesini G. Pilot study on the additive effects of berberine and oral type 2 diabetes agents for patients with suboptimal glycemic

control. Diabetes Metab Syndr Obes 2012; 5: 213-7.
[http://dx.doi.org/10.2147/DMSO.S33718] [PMID: 22924000]

[46]   Di Pierro F, Putignano P, Villanova N, Montesi L, Moscatiello S, Marchesini G. Preliminary study about the possible glycemic clinical advantage in using a fixed combination of *Berberis aristata* and *Silybum marianum* standardized extracts *versus* only *Berberis aristata* in patients with type 2 diabetes. Clin Pharmacol 2013; 5: 167-74.
[http://dx.doi.org/10.2147/CPAA.S54308] [PMID: 24277991]

[47]   Di Pierro F, Bellone I, Rapacioli G, Putignano P. Clinical role of a fixed combination of standardized *Berberis aristata* and *Silybum marianum* extracts in diabetic and hypercholesterolemic patients intolerant to statins. Diabetes Metab Syndr Obes 2015; 8: 89-96.
[http://dx.doi.org/10.2147/DMSO.S78877] [PMID: 25678808]

[48]   Akhtar MS, Athar MA, Yaqub M. Effect of *Momordica charantia* on blood glucose level of normal and alloxan-diabetic rabbits. Planta Med 1981; 42(3): 205-12.
[http://dx.doi.org/10.1055/s-2007-971629] [PMID: 7280086]

[49]   Welihinda J, Karunanayake EH, Sheriff MH, Jayasinghe KS. Effect of *Momordica charantia* on the glucose tolerance in maturity onset diabetes. J Ethnopharmacol 1986; 17(3): 277-82.
[http://dx.doi.org/10.1016/0378-8741(86)90116-9] [PMID: 3807390]

[50]   Baldwa VS, Bhandari CM, Pangaria A, Goyal RK. Clinical trial in patients with diabetes mellitus of an insulin-like compound obtained from plant source. Ups J Med Sci 1977; 82(1): 39-41.
[http://dx.doi.org/10.3109/03009737709179057] [PMID: 20078273]

[51]   Fuangchan A, Sonthisombat P, Seubnukarn T, *et al.* Hypoglycemic effect of bitter melon compared with metformin in newly diagnosed type 2 diabetes patients. J Ethnopharmacol 2011; 134(2): 422-8.
[http://dx.doi.org/10.1016/j.jep.2010.12.045] [PMID: 21211558]

[52]   Krawinkel MB, Ludwig C, Swai ME, Yang RY, Chun KP, Habicht SD. Bitter gourd reduces elevated fasting plasma glucose levels in an intervention study among prediabetics in Tanzania. J Ethnopharmacol 2018; 216: 1-7.
[http://dx.doi.org/10.1016/j.jep.2018.01.016] [PMID: 29339109]

[53]   Capaldo B, Napoli R, Di Bonito P, Albano G, Saccà L. Carnitine improves peripheral glucose disposal in non-insulin-dependent diabetic patients. Diabetes Res Clin Pract 1991; 14(3): 191-5.
[http://dx.doi.org/10.1016/0168-8227(91)90020-E] [PMID: 1778112]

[54]   Giancaterini A, De Gaetano A, Mingrone G, *et al.* Acetyl-L-carnitine infusion increases glucose disposal in type 2 diabetic patients. Metabolism 2000; 49(6): 704-8.
[http://dx.doi.org/10.1053/meta.2000.6250] [PMID: 10877193]

[55]   Mingrone G, Greco AV, Capristo E, *et al.* L-carnitine improves glucose disposal in type 2 diabetic patients. J Am Coll Nutr 1999; 18(1): 77-82.
[http://dx.doi.org/10.1080/07315724.1999.10718830] [PMID: 10067662]

[56]   Mirfeizi M, Mehdizadeh Tourzani Z, Mirfeizi SZ, Asghari Jafarabadi M, Rezvani HR, Afzali M. Controlling type 2 diabetes mellitus with herbal medicines: A triple-blind randomized clinical trial of efficacy and safety. J Diabetes 2016; 8(5): 647-56.
[http://dx.doi.org/10.1111/1753-0407.12342] [PMID: 26362826]

[57]   Yusni Y, Zufry H, Meutia F, Sucipto KW. The effects of celery leaf (*apium graveolens* L.) treatment on blood glucose and insulin levels in elderly pre-diabetics. Saudi Med J 2018; 39(2): 154-60.
[http://dx.doi.org/10.15537/smj.2018.2.21238] [PMID: 29436564]

[58]   Lee NA, Reasner CA. Beneficial effect of chromium supplementation on serum triglyceride levels in NIDDM. Diabetes Care 1994; 17(12): 1449-52.
[http://dx.doi.org/10.2337/diacare.17.12.1449] [PMID: 7882815]

[59]   Anderson RA, Cheng N, Bryden NA, *et al.* Elevated intakes of supplemental chromium improve glucose and insulin variables in individuals with type 2 diabetes. Diabetes 1997; 46(11): 1786-91.

[http://dx.doi.org/10.2337/diab.46.11.1786] [PMID: 9356027]

[60] Cefalu WT, Bell-Farrow AD, Stegner J, *et al.* Effect of chromium picolinate on insulin sensitivity *in vivo.* Journal of Trace Elements in Experimental Medicine: The Official Publication of the International Society for Trace Element Research in Humans 1999; 12(2): 71-83.
[http://dx.doi.org/10.1002/(SICI)1520-670X(1999)12:2<71::AID-JTRA4>3.0.CO;2-8]

[61] Bahijiri SM, Mira SA, Mufti AM, Ajabnoor MA. The effects of inorganic chromium and brewer's yeast supplementation on glucose tolerance, serum lipids and drug dosage in individuals with type 2 diabetes. Saudi Med J 2000; 21(9): 831-7.
[PMID: 11376359]

[62] Uusitupa MI, Mykkänen L, Siitonen O, *et al.* Chromium supplementation in impaired glucose tolerance of elderly: effects on blood glucose, plasma insulin, C-peptide and lipid levels. Br J Nutr 1992; 68(1): 209-16.
[http://dx.doi.org/10.1079/BJN19920078] [PMID: 1390605]

[63] Anderson RA, Polansky MM, Bryden NA, Canary JJ. Supplemental-chromium effects on glucose, insulin, glucagon, and urinary chromium losses in subjects consuming controlled low-chromium diets. Am J Clin Nutr 1991; 54(5): 909-16.
[http://dx.doi.org/10.1093/ajcn/54.5.909] [PMID: 1951165]

[64] Abraham AS, Brooks BA, Eylath U. The effects of chromium supplementation on serum glucose and lipids in patients with and without non-insulin-dependent diabetes. Metabolism 1992; 41(7): 768-71.
[http://dx.doi.org/10.1016/0026-0495(92)90318-5] [PMID: 1619996]

[65] Anderson RA, Roussel AM, Zouari N, Mahjoub S, Matheau JM, Kerkeni A. Potential antioxidant effects of zinc and chromium supplementation in people with type 2 diabetes mellitus. J Am Coll Nutr 2001; 20(3): 212-8.
[http://dx.doi.org/10.1080/07315724.2001.10719034] [PMID: 11444416]

[66] Allen RW, Schwartzman E, Baker WL, Coleman CI, Phung OJ. Cinnamon use in type 2 diabetes: an updated systematic review and meta-analysis. Ann Fam Med 2013; 11(5): 452-9. t
[http://dx.doi.org/10.1370/afm.1517] [PMID: 24019277]

[67] Mang B, Wolters M, Schmitt B, *et al.* Effects of a cinnamon extract on plasma glucose, HbA, and serum lipids in diabetes mellitus type 2. Eur J Clin Invest 2006; 36(5): 340-4.
[http://dx.doi.org/10.1111/j.1365-2362.2006.01629.x] [PMID: 16634838]

[68] Azad Khan AK, Akhtar S, Mahtab H. *Coccinia indica* in the treatment of patients with diabetes mellitus. Bangladesh Med Res Counc Bull 1979; 5(2): 60-6.
[PMID: 399436]

[69] Kamble SM, Jyotishi GS, Kamlakar PL, Vaidya SM. Efficacy of *Coccinia indica* W. &A in diabetes mellitus. J Res Ayurveda Siddha 1996; 17: 77-84.

[70] Kamble SM, Kamlakar PL, Vaidya S, Bambole VD. Influence of *Coccinia indica* on certain enzymes in glycolytic and lipolytic pathway in human diabetes. Indian J Med Sci 1998; 52(4): 143-6.
[PMID: 9770877]

[71] Hanai H, Ikuma M, Sato Y, *et al.* Long-term effects of water-soluble corn bran hemicellulose on glucose tolerance in obese and non-obese patients: improved insulin sensitivity and glucose metabolism in obese subjects. Biosci Biotechnol Biochem 1997; 61(8): 1358-61.
[http://dx.doi.org/10.1271/bbb.61.1358] [PMID: 9301120]

[72] Usharani P, Mateen AA, Naidu MU, Raju YS, Chandra N. Effect of NCB-02, atorvastatin and placebo on endothelial function, oxidative stress and inflammatory markers in patients with type 2 diabetes mellitus: a randomized, parallel-group, placebo-controlled, 8-week study. Drugs R D 2008; 9(4): 243-50.
[http://dx.doi.org/10.2165/00126839-200809040-00004] [PMID: 18588355]

[73] Na LX, Li Y, Pan HZ, *et al.* Curcuminoids exert glucose-lowering effect in type 2 diabetes by

decreasing serum free fatty acids: a double-blind, placebo-controlled trial. Mol Nutr Food Res 2013; 57(9): 1569-77.
[http://dx.doi.org/10.1002/mnfr.201200131] [PMID: 22930403]

[74]   Rahimi HR, Mohammadpour AH, Dastani M, *et al.* The effect of nano-curcumin on HbA1c, fasting blood glucose, and lipid profile in diabetic subjects: a randomized clinical trial. Avicenna J Phytomed 2016; 6(5): 567-77.
[PMID: 27761427]

[75]   Panahi Y, Khalili N, Sahebi E, *et al.* Curcuminoids modify lipid profile in type 2 diabetes mellitus: A randomized controlled trial. Complement Ther Med 2017; 33: 1-5.
[http://dx.doi.org/10.1016/j.ctim.2017.05.006] [PMID: 28735818]

[76]   Sarker MMR, Tandra TH, Akhter S, Muse JS. Antidiabetic potential of a novel formulation of functional foods in patients with type 2 diabetes mellitus: a single centre, single blind, prospective interventional study. Research Updates in Medical Science 2019; 7 (Suppl. 1): 3.

[77]   Sharma RD, Raghuram TC. Hypoglycaemic effect of fenugreek seeds in non-insulin dependent diabetic subjects. Nutr Res 1990; 10(7): 731-9.
[http://dx.doi.org/10.1016/S0271-5317(05)80822-X]

[78]   Sharma RD, Raghuram TC, Rao NS. Effect of fenugreek seeds on blood glucose and serum lipids in type I diabetes. Eur J Clin Nutr 1990; 44(4): 301-6.
[PMID: 2194788]

[79]   Sharma RD. Effect of fenugreek seeds and leaves on blood glucose and serum insulin responses in human subjects. Nutr Res 1986; 6(12): 1353-64.
[http://dx.doi.org/10.1016/S0271-5317(86)80020-3]

[80]   Madar Z, Abel R, Samish S, Arad J. Glucose-lowering effect of fenugreek in non-insulin dependent diabetics. Eur J Clin Nutr 1988; 42(1): 51-4.
[PMID: 3286242]

[81]   Lu FR, Shen L, Qin Y, Gao L, Li H, Dai Y. Clinical observation on *Trigonella foenum-graecum* L. total saponins in combination with sulfonylureas in the treatment of type 2 diabetes mellitus. Chin J Integr Med 2008; 14(1): 56-60.
[http://dx.doi.org/10.1007/s11655-007-9005-3] [PMID: 18219452]

[82]   Serraclara A, Hawkins F, Pérez C, Domínguez E, Campillo JE, Torres MD. Hypoglycemic action of an oral fig-leaf decoction in type-I diabetic patients. Diabetes Res Clin Pract 1998; 39(1): 19-22.
[http://dx.doi.org/10.1016/S0168-8227(97)00112-5] [PMID: 9597370]

[83]   Ryuk JA, Lixia M, Cao S, Ko BS, Park S. Efficacy and safety of Gegen Qinlian decoction for normalizing hyperglycemia in diabetic patients: A systematic review and meta-analysis of randomized clinical trials. Complement Ther Med 2017; 33: 6-13.
[http://dx.doi.org/10.1016/j.ctim.2017.05.004] [PMID: 28735827]

[84]   Bauer PV, Duca FA. Targeting the gastrointestinal tract to treat type 2 diabetes. J Endocrinol 2016; 230(3): R95-R113.
[http://dx.doi.org/10.1530/JOE-16-0056] [PMID: 27496374]

[85]   Goulet O. Potential role of the intestinal microbiota in programming health and disease. Nutrition reviews 2015; 73(suppl_1): 32-40.
[http://dx.doi.org/10.1093/nutrit/nuv039]

[86]   Zemestani M, Rafraf M, Asghari-Jafarabadi M. Chamomile tea improves glycemic indices and antioxidants status in patients with type 2 diabetes mellitus. Nutrition 2016; 32(1): 66-72.
[http://dx.doi.org/10.1016/j.nut.2015.07.011] [PMID: 26437613]

[87]   Sotaniemi EA, Haapakoski E, Rautio A. Ginseng therapy in non-insulin-dependent diabetic patients. Diabetes Care 1995; 18(10): 1373-5.
[http://dx.doi.org/10.2337/diacare.18.10.1373] [PMID: 8721940]

[88]   Vuksan V, Sievenpiper JL, Koo VY, *et al.* American ginseng (*Panax quinquefolius* L) reduces postprandial glycemia in nondiabetic subjects and subjects with type 2 diabetes mellitus. Arch Intern Med 2000; 160(7): 1009-13.
       [http://dx.doi.org/10.1001/archinte.160.7.1009] [PMID: 10761967]

[89]   Feinberg T, Wieland LS, Miller LE, *et al.* Polyherbal dietary supplementation for prediabetic adults: study protocol for a randomized controlled trial. Trials 2019; 20(1): 24.
       [http://dx.doi.org/10.1186/s13063-018-3032-6] [PMID: 30616613]

[90]   Yang X, Kong F. Evaluation of the *in vitro* α-glucosidase inhibitory activity of green tea polyphenols and different tea types. J Sci Food Agric 2016; 96(3): 777-82.
       [http://dx.doi.org/10.1002/jsfa.7147] [PMID: 25707691]

[91]   Nagao T, Meguro S, Hase T, *et al.* A catechin-rich beverage improves obesity and blood glucose control in patients with type 2 diabetes. Obesity (Silver Spring) 2009; 17(2): 310-7.
       [http://dx.doi.org/10.1038/oby.2008.505] [PMID: 19008868]

[92]   Nahas R, Moher M. Complementary and alternative medicine for the treatment of type 2 diabetes. Can Fam Physician 2009; 55(6): 591-6.
       [PMID: 19509199]

[93]   Kumar SN, Mani UV, Mani I. An open label study on the supplementation of *Gymnema sylvestre* in type 2 diabetics. J Diet Suppl 2010; 7(3): 273-82.
       [http://dx.doi.org/10.3109/19390211.2010.505901] [PMID: 22432517]

[94]   Baskaran K, Kizar Ahamath B, Radha Shanmugasundaram K, Shanmugasundaram ER. Antidiabetic effect of a leaf extract from *Gymnema sylvestre* in non-insulin-dependent diabetes mellitus patients. J Ethnopharmacol 1990; 30(3): 295-300.
       [http://dx.doi.org/10.1016/0378-8741(90)90108-6] [PMID: 2259217]

[95]   Shanmugasundaram ER, Rajeswari G, Baskaran K, Rajesh Kumar BR, Radha Shanmugasundaram K, Kizar Ahmath B. Use of *Gymnema sylvestre* leaf extract in the control of blood glucose in insulin-dependent diabetes mellitus. J Ethnopharmacol 1990; 30(3): 281-94.
       [http://dx.doi.org/10.1016/0378-8741(90)90107-5] [PMID: 2259216]

[96]   Obara K, Mizutani M, Hitomi Y, Yajima H, Kondo K. Isohumulones, the bitter component of beer, improve hyperglycemia and decrease body fat in Japanese subjects with prediabetes. Clin Nutr 2009; 28(3): 278-84.
       [http://dx.doi.org/10.1016/j.clnu.2009.03.012] [PMID: 19395131]

[97]   Pan A, Sun J, Chen Y, *et al.* Effects of a flaxseed-derived lignan supplement in type 2 diabetic patients: a randomized, double-blind, cross-over trial. PLoS One 2007; 2(11)e1148
       [http://dx.doi.org/10.1371/journal.pone.0001148] [PMID: 17987126]

[98]   de Lordes Lima M, Cruz T, Pousada JC, Rodrigues LE, Barbosa K, Canguçu V. The effect of magnesium supplementation in increasing doses on the control of type 2 diabetes. Diabetes Care 1998; 21(5): 682-6.
       [http://dx.doi.org/10.2337/diacare.21.5.682] [PMID: 9589224]

[99]   Eibl NL, Kopp HP, Nowak HR, Schnack CJ, Hopmeier PG, Schernthaner G. Hypomagnesemia in type II diabetes: effect of a 3-month replacement therapy. Diabetes Care 1995; 18(2): 188-92.
       [http://dx.doi.org/10.2337/diacare.18.2.188] [PMID: 7729296]

[100] Paolisso G, Sgambato S, Gambardella A, *et al.* Daily magnesium supplements improve glucose handling in elderly subjects. Am J Clin Nutr 1992; 55(6): 1161-7.
       [http://dx.doi.org/10.1093/ajcn/55.6.1161] [PMID: 1595589]

[101] de Valk HW, Verkaaik R, van Rijn HJ, Geerdink RA, Struyvenberg A. Oral magnesium supplementation in insulin-requiring Type 2 diabetic patients. Diabet Med 1998; 15(6): 503-7.
       [http://dx.doi.org/10.1002/(SICI)1096-9136(199806)15:6<503::AID-DIA596>3.0.CO;2-M] [PMID: 9632126]

[102]   Paolisso G, Scheen A, Cozzolino D, *et al.* Changes in glucose turnover parameters and improvement of glucose oxidation after 4-week magnesium administration in elderly noninsulin-dependent (type II) diabetic patients. J Clin Endocrinol Metab 1994; 78(6): 1510-4.
[PMID: 8200955]

[103]   Paolisso G, Sgambato S, Pizza G, Passariello N, Varricchio M, D'Onofrio F. Improved insulin response and action by chronic magnesium administration in aged NIDDM subjects. Diabetes Care 1989; 12(4): 265-9.
[http://dx.doi.org/10.2337/diacare.12.4.265] [PMID: 2651054]

[104]   Nayebi N, Esteghamati A, Meysamie A, *et al.* The effects of a *Melissa officinalis* L. based product on metabolic parameters in patients with type 2 diabetes mellitus: A randomized double-blinded controlled clinical trial. J Complement Integr Med 2019; 16(3): /j/jcim.2019.16.issue-3/jcim-20-8-0088/jcim-2018-0088.xml.
[http://dx.doi.org/10.1515/jcim-2018-0088] [PMID: 30681971]

[105]   Velussi M, Cernigoi AM, De Monte A, Dapas F, Caffau C, Zilli M. Long-term (12 months) treatment with an anti-oxidant drug (silymarin) is effective on hyperinsulinemia, exogenous insulin need and malondialdehyde levels in cirrhotic diabetic patients. J Hepatol 1997; 26(4): 871-9.
[http://dx.doi.org/10.1016/S0168-8278(97)80255-3] [PMID: 9126802]

[106]   Huseini HF, Larijani B, Heshmat R, *et al.* The efficacy of *Silybum marianum* (L.) Gaertn. (silymarin) in the treatment of type II diabetes: a randomized, double-blind, placebo-controlled, clinical trial. Phytother Res 2006; 20(12): 1036-9.
[http://dx.doi.org/10.1002/ptr.1988] [PMID: 17072885]

[107]   Hussain SA. Silymarin as an adjunct to glibenclamide therapy improves long-term and postprandial glycemic control and body mass index in type 2 diabetes. J Med Food 2007; 10(3): 543-7.
[http://dx.doi.org/10.1089/jmf.2006.089] [PMID: 17887949]

[108]   Ramezani MA, Azarabadi M, Abdi H, Baher G, Huseini M. The effects of *Silybum marianum* (L.) Gaertn. seed extract on glycemic control in type II diabetic patient's candidate for insulin therapy visiting endocrinology clinic in baqiyatallah hospital in the years of 2006. Faslnamah-i Giyahan-i Daruyi 2008; 2(26): 79-84.

[109]   Mohammadi SM, Afkhami Ardacani M, Salami MS, Bolurani S. Effects of silymarin on insulin resistance and blood lipid profile in first-degree relatives of type 2 diabetic patients. Faslnamah-i Giyahan-i Daruyi 2013; 2(46): 170-6.

[110]   Russo EM, Reichelt AA, De-Sá JR, *et al.* Clinical trial of *Myrcia uniflora* and *Bauhinia forficata* leaf extracts in normal and diabetic patients. Braz J Med Biol Res 1990; 23(1): 11-20.
[PMID: 2201413]

[111]   Daryabeygi-Khotbehsara R, Golzarand M, Ghaffari MP, Djafarian K. *Nigella sativa* improves glucose homeostasis and serum lipids in type 2 diabetes: A systematic review and meta-analysis. Complement Ther Med 2017; 35: 6-13.
[http://dx.doi.org/10.1016/j.ctim.2017.08.016] [PMID: 29154069]

[112]   Alimohammadi S, Hobbenaghi R, Javanbakht J, *et al.* Protective and antidiabetic effects of extract from *Nigella sativa* on blood glucose concentrations against streptozotocin (STZ)-induced diabetic in rats: an experimental study with histopathological evaluation. Diagn Pathol 2013; 8(1): 137.
[http://dx.doi.org/10.1186/1746-1596-8-137] [PMID: 23947821]

[113]   Heshmati J, Namazi N, Memarzadeh MR, Taghizadeh M, Kolahdooz F. *Nigella sativa* oil affects glucose metabolism and lipid concentrations in patients with type 2 diabetes: A randomized, double-blind, placebo-controlled trial. Food Res Int 2015; 70: 87-93.
[http://dx.doi.org/10.1016/j.foodres.2015.01.030]

[114]   Kanter M, Meral I, Yener Z, Ozbek H, Demir H. Partial regeneration/proliferation of the β-cells in the islets of Langerhans by *Nigella sativa* L. in streptozotocin-induced diabetic rats. Tohoku J Exp Med 2003; 201(4): 213-9.

[http://dx.doi.org/10.1620/tjem.201.213] [PMID: 14690013]

[115] Fararh KM, Atoji Y, Shimizu Y, Shiina T, Nikami H, Takewaki T. Mechanisms of the hypoglycaemic and immunopotentiating effects of *Nigella sativa* L. oil in streptozotocin-induced diabetic hamsters. Res Vet Sci 2004; 77(2): 123-9.
[http://dx.doi.org/10.1016/j.rvsc.2004.03.002] [PMID: 15196902]

[116] Benhaddou-Andaloussi A, Martineau LC, Spoor D, *et al.* Antidiabetic activity of *Nigella sativa*. Seed extract in cultured pancreatic β-cells, skeletal muscle cells, and adipocytes. Pharm Biol 2008; 46(1-2): 96-104.
[http://dx.doi.org/10.1080/13880200701734810]

[117] Benhaddou-Andaloussi A, Martineau L, Vuong T, *et al.* The *in vivo* antidiabetic activity of *Nigella sativa* is mediated through activation of the AMPK pathway and increased muscle Glut4 content. Evidence-Based Complementary and Alternative Medicine 2011; 2011

[118] Fararh KM, Ibrahim AK, Elsonosy YA. Thymoquinone enhances the activities of enzymes related to energy metabolism in peripheral leukocytes of diabetic rats. Res Vet Sci 2010; 88(3): 400-4.
[http://dx.doi.org/10.1016/j.rvsc.2009.10.008] [PMID: 19931880]

[119] Augusti KT, Benaim ME. Effect of essential oil of onion (allyl propyl disulphide) on blood glucose, free fatty acid and insulin levels of normal subjects. Clin Chim Acta 1975; 60(1): 121-3.
[http://dx.doi.org/10.1016/0009-8981(75)90190-4] [PMID: 1126028]

[120] Frati AC, Gordillo BE, Altamirano P, Ariza CR, Cortés-Franco R, Chavez-Negrete A. Acute hypoglycemic effect of *Opuntia streptacantha* Lemaire in NIDDM. Diabetes Care 1990; 13(4): 455-6.
[http://dx.doi.org/10.2337/diacare.13.4.455] [PMID: 2318110]

[121] Frati AC, Xilotl Díaz N, Altamirano P, Ariza R, López-Ledesma R. The effect of two sequential doses of *Opuntia streptacantha* upon glycemia. Arch Invest Med (Mex) 1991; 22(3-4): 333-6.
[PMID: 1844121]

[122] Liu X, Wei J, Tan F, Zhou S, Würthwein G, Rohdewald P. Antidiabetic effect of Pycnogenol French maritime pine bark extract in patients with diabetes type II. Life Sci 2004; 75(21): 2505-13.
[http://dx.doi.org/10.1016/j.lfs.2003.10.043] [PMID: 15363656]

[123] Liu X, Zhou HJ, Rohdewald P. French maritime pine bark extract Pycnogenol dose-dependently lowers glucose in type 2 diabetic patients. Diabetes Care 2004; 27(3): 839.
[http://dx.doi.org/10.2337/diacare.27.3.839] [PMID: 14988316]

[124] Zibadi S, Rohdewald PJ, Park D, Watson RR. Reduction of cardiovascular risk factors in subjects with type 2 diabetes by Pycnogenol supplementation. Nutr Res 2008; 28(5): 315-20.
[http://dx.doi.org/10.1016/j.nutres.2008.03.003] [PMID: 19083426]

[125] Howes JB, Tran D, Brillante D, Howes LG. Effects of dietary supplementation with isoflavones from red clover on ambulatory blood pressure and endothelial function in postmenopausal type 2 diabetes. Diabetes Obes Metab 2003; 5(5): 325-32.
[http://dx.doi.org/10.1046/j.1463-1326.2003.00282.x] [PMID: 12940870]

[126] Bhatt JK, Thomas S, Nanjan MJ. Resveratrol supplementation improves glycemic control in type 2 diabetes mellitus. Nutr Res 2012; 32(7): 537-41.
[http://dx.doi.org/10.1016/j.nutres.2012.06.003] [PMID: 22901562]

[127] Movahed A, Nabipour I, Lieben Louis X, *et al.* Antihyperglycemic effects of short term resveratrol supplementation in type 2 diabetic patients. Evid Based Complement Alternat Med 2013; 2013851267
[http://dx.doi.org/10.1155/2013/851267] [PMID: 24073011]

[128] Witte AV, Kerti L, Margulies DS, Flöel A. Effects of resveratrol on memory performance, hippocampal functional connectivity, and glucose metabolism in healthy older adults. J Neurosci 2014; 34(23): 7862-70.
[http://dx.doi.org/10.1523/JNEUROSCI.0385-14.2014] [PMID: 24899709]

[129] Senadheera SP, Ekanayake S, Wanigatunge C. Anti-hyperglycaemic effects of herbal porridge made

of *Scoparia dulcis* leaf extract in diabetics - a randomized crossover clinical trial. BMC Complement Altern Med 2015; 15(1): 410.
[http://dx.doi.org/10.1186/s12906-015-0935-6] [PMID: 26582144]

[130]   Xiong MQ, Liang LW, Lin AZ, *et al.* Clinical and experimental study of Persical Decoction for Purgation with Addition in the treatment of non-insulin dependent diabetes mellitus. Chinese Journal of Integrated Traditional and Western Medicine 1995; 1(2): 96-9.

[131]   Kim JI, Kim JC, Kang MJ, Lee MS, Kim JJ, Cha IJ. Effects of pinitol isolated from soybeans on glycaemic control and cardiovascular risk factors in Korean patients with type II diabetes mellitus: a randomized controlled study. Eur J Clin Nutr 2005; 59(3): 456-8.
[http://dx.doi.org/10.1038/sj.ejcn.1602081] [PMID: 15536472]

[132]   Barriocanal LA, Palacios M, Benitez G, *et al.* Apparent lack of pharmacological effect of steviol glycosides used as sweeteners in humans. A pilot study of repeated exposures in some normotensive and hypotensive individuals and in Type 1 and Type 2 diabetics. Regul Toxicol Pharmacol 2008; 51(1): 37-41.
[http://dx.doi.org/10.1016/j.yrtph.2008.02.006] [PMID: 18397817]

[133]   Yeh GY, Eisenberg DM, Kaptchuk TJ, Phillips RS. Systematic review of herbs and dietary supplements for glycemic control in diabetes. Diabetes Care 2003; 26(4): 1277-94.
[http://dx.doi.org/10.2337/diacare.26.4.1277] [PMID: 12663610]

[134]   Namdul T, Sood A, Ramakrishnan L, Pandey RM, Moorthy D. Efficacy of Tibetan medicine as an adjunct in the treatment of type 2 diabetes. Diabetes Care 2001; 24(1): 175-6.
[http://dx.doi.org/10.2337/diacare.24.1.176] [PMID: 11194229]

[135]   Vray M, Attali JR. Chinese-French Scientific Committee for the Study of Diabetes. Randomized study of glibenclamide *versus* traditional Chinese treatment in type 2 diabetic patients. Diabete Metab 1995; 21(6): 433-9.
[PMID: 8593925]

[136]   Agrawal P, Rai V, Singh RB. Randomized placebo-controlled, single blind trial of holy basil leaves in patients with noninsulin-dependent diabetes mellitus. Int J Clin Pharmacol Ther 1996; 34(9): 406-9.
[PMID: 8880292]

[137]   Cheng SH, Ismail A, Anthony J, Ng OC, Hamid AA, Barakatun-Nisak MY. Eight weeks of *Cosmos caudatus* (Ulam Raja) supplementation improves glycemic status in patients with type 2 diabetes: a randomized controlled trial. Evidence-Based Complementary and Alternative Medicine 2015.2015.

[138]   Cohen N, Halberstam M, Shlimovich P, Chang CJ, Shamoon H, Rossetti L. Oral vanadyl sulfate improves hepatic and peripheral insulin sensitivity in patients with non-insulin-dependent diabetes mellitus. J Clin Invest 1995; 95(6): 2501-9.
[http://dx.doi.org/10.1172/JCI117951] [PMID: 7769096]

[139]   Halberstam M, Cohen N, Shlimovich P, Rossetti L, Shamoon H. Oral vanadyl sulfate improves insulin sensitivity in NIDDM but not in obese nondiabetic subjects. Diabetes 1996; 45(5): 659-66.
[http://dx.doi.org/10.2337/diab.45.5.659] [PMID: 8621019]

[140]   Boden G, Chen X, Ruiz J, van Rossum GD, Turco S. Effects of vanadyl sulfate on carbohydrate and lipid metabolism in patients with non-insulin-dependent diabetes mellitus. Metabolism 1996; 45(9): 1130-5.
[http://dx.doi.org/10.1016/S0026-0495(96)90013-X] [PMID: 8781301]

[141]   Cusi K, Cukier S, DeFronzo RA, Torres M, Puchulu FM, Redondo JC. Vanadyl sulfate improves hepatic and muscle insulin sensitivity in type 2 diabetes. J Clin Endocrinol Metab 2001; 86(3): 1410-7.
[http://dx.doi.org/10.1210/jc.86.3.1410] [PMID: 11238540]

[142]   Goldfine AB, Simonson DC, Folli F, Patti ME, Kahn CR. Metabolic effects of sodium metavanadate in humans with insulin-dependent and noninsulin-dependent diabetes mellitus *in vivo* and *in vitro* studies. J Clin Endocrinol Metab 1995; 80(11): 3311-20.
[PMID: 7593444]

[143] Goldwaser I, Gefel D, Gershonov E, Fridkin M, Shechter Y. Insulin-like effects of vanadium: basic and clinical implications. J Inorg Biochem 2000; 80(1-2): 21-5.
[http://dx.doi.org/10.1016/S0162-0134(00)00035-0] [PMID: 10885459]

[144] Frei B, Stocker R, Ames BN. Antioxidant defenses and lipid peroxidation in human blood plasma. Proc Natl Acad Sci USA 1988; 85(24): 9748-52.
[http://dx.doi.org/10.1073/pnas.85.24.9748] [PMID: 3200852]

[145] Frei B, England L, Ames BN. Ascorbate is an outstanding antioxidant in human blood plasma. Proc Natl Acad Sci USA 1989; 86(16): 6377-81.
[http://dx.doi.org/10.1073/pnas.86.16.6377] [PMID: 2762330]

[146] Retsky KL, Freeman MW, Frei B. Ascorbic acid oxidation product(s) protect human low density lipoprotein against atherogenic modification. Anti- rather than prooxidant activity of vitamin C in the presence of transition metal ions. J Biol Chem 1993; 268(2): 1304-9.
[PMID: 8419332]

[147] Chen MS, Hutchinson ML, Pecoraro RE, Lee WY, Labbé RF. Hyperglycemia-induced intracellular depletion of ascorbic acid in human mononuclear leukocytes. Diabetes 1983; 32(11): 1078-81.
[http://dx.doi.org/10.2337/diab.32.11.1078] [PMID: 6357907]

[148] Yue DK, McLennan S, Fisher E, *et al.* Ascorbic acid metabolism and polyol pathway in diabetes. Diabetes 1989; 38(2): 257-61.
[http://dx.doi.org/10.2337/diab.38.2.257] [PMID: 2492477]

[149] Cunningham JJ, Ellis SL, McVeigh KL, Levine RE, Calles-Escandon J. Reduced mononuclear leukocyte ascorbic acid content in adults with insulin-dependent diabetes mellitus consuming adequate dietary vitamin C. Metabolism 1991; 40(2): 146-9.
[http://dx.doi.org/10.1016/0026-0495(91)90165-S] [PMID: 1988772]

[150] Ting HH, Timimi FK, Boles KS, Creager SJ, Ganz P, Creager MA. Vitamin C improves endothelium-dependent vasodilation in patients with non-insulin-dependent diabetes mellitus. J Clin Invest 1996; 97(1): 22-8.
[http://dx.doi.org/10.1172/JCI118394] [PMID: 8550838]

[151] Paolisso G, D'Amore A, Balbi V, *et al.* Plasma vitamin C affects glucose homeostasis in healthy subjects and in non-insulin-dependent diabetics. Am J Physiol 1994; 266(2 Pt 1): E261-8.
[PMID: 8141285]

[152] Paolisso G, D'Amore A, Giugliano D, Ceriello A, Varricchio M, D'Onofrio F. Pharmacologic doses of vitamin E improve insulin action in healthy subjects and non-insulin-dependent diabetic patients. Am J Clin Nutr 1993; 57(5): 650-6.
[http://dx.doi.org/10.1093/ajcn/57.5.650] [PMID: 8480681]

[153] Reaven PD, Herold DA, Barnett J, Edelman S. Effects of Vitamin E on susceptibility of low-density lipoprotein and low-density lipoprotein subfractions to oxidation and on protein glycation in NIDDM. Diabetes Care 1995; 18(6): 807-16.
[http://dx.doi.org/10.2337/diacare.18.6.807] [PMID: 7555507]

[154] Ceriello A, Giugliano D, Quatraro A, Donzella C, Dipalo G, Lefebvre PJ. Vitamin E reduction of protein glycosylation in diabetes. New prospect for prevention of diabetic complications? Diabetes Care 1991; 14(1): 68-72.
[http://dx.doi.org/10.2337/diacare.14.1.68] [PMID: 1991440]

[155] Paolisso G, D'Amore A, Galzerano D, *et al.* Daily vitamin E supplements improve metabolic control but not insulin secretion in elderly type II diabetic patients. Diabetes Care 1993; 16(11): 1433-7.
[http://dx.doi.org/10.2337/diacare.16.11.1433] [PMID: 8299431]

[156] Gómez-Pérez FJ, Valles-Sánchez VE, López-Alvarenga JC, *et al.* Vitamin E modifies neither fructosamine nor HbA1c levels in poorly controlled diabetes. Revista de investigacion clinica; organo del Hospital de Enfermedades de la Nutricion 1996; 48(6): 421-4.

[157] Jain SK, McVie R, Jaramillo JJ, Palmer M, Smith T. Effect of modest vitamin E supplementation on blood glycated hemoglobin and triglyceride levels and red cell indices in type I diabetic patients. J Am Coll Nutr 1996; 15(5): 458-61.
[http://dx.doi.org/10.1080/07315724.1996.10718624] [PMID: 8892171]

[158] Zibaeenezhad MJ, Farhadi P, Attar A, Mosleh A, Amirmoezi F, Azimi A. Effects of walnut oil on lipid profiles in hyperlipidemic type 2 diabetic patients: a randomized, double-blind, placebo-controlled trial. Nutr Diabetes 2017; 7(4): e259.
[http://dx.doi.org/10.1038/nutd.2017.8] [PMID: 28394361]

[159] Asai A, Nakagawa K, Higuchi O, *et al.* Effect of mulberry leaf extract with enriched 1-deoxynojirimycin content on postprandial glycemic control in subjects with impaired glucose metabolism. J Diabetes Investig 2011; 2(4): 318-23.
[http://dx.doi.org/10.1111/j.2040-1124.2011.00101.x] [PMID: 24843505]

[160] Ji L, Tong X, Wang H, *et al.* Evidence-Based Medical Research of Xiaoke Pill Study Group. Efficacy and safety of traditional chinese medicine for diabetes: a double-blind, randomised, controlled trial. PLoS One 2013; 8(2): e56703.
[http://dx.doi.org/10.1371/journal.pone.0056703] [PMID: 23460810]

[161] Maritim AC, Sanders RA, Watkins JB III. Diabetes, oxidative stress, and antioxidants: a review. J Biochem Mol Toxicol 2003; 17(1): 24-38.
[http://dx.doi.org/10.1002/jbt.10058] [PMID: 12616644]

[162] Ceriello A, Motz E. Is oxidative stress the pathogenic mechanism underlying insulin resistance, diabetes, and cardiovascular disease? The common soil hypothesis revisited. Arterioscler Thromb Vasc Biol 2004; 24(5): 816-23.
[http://dx.doi.org/10.1161/01.ATV.0000122852.22604.78] [PMID: 14976002]

[163] Valko M, Leibfritz D, Moncol J, Cronin MTD, Mazur M, Telser J. Free radicals and antioxidants in normal physiological functions and human disease. Int J Biochem Cell Biol 2007; 39(1): 44-84.
[http://dx.doi.org/10.1016/j.biocel.2006.07.001] [PMID: 16978905]

[164] Evans JL, Maddux BA, Goldfine ID. The molecular basis for oxidative stress-induced insulin resistance. Antioxid Redox Signal 2005; 7(7-8): 1040-52.
[http://dx.doi.org/10.1089/ars.2005.7.1040] [PMID: 15998259]

CHAPTER 2

Curcumin: A Drug of Choice for the Treatment of Diabetes and Hypertension

Adeeb Shehzad[1], Raheem Shahzad[2], Meneerah A. Aljafary[3] and Ebtesam A. Al-Suhaimi[*,3,4]

[1] *Department of Pharmacy, Institute for Research and Medical Consultations, Imam Abdulrahman Bin Faisal University, Dammam, Saudi Arabia*

[2] *Department of Horticulture, University of Haripur, Haripur, Pakistan*

[3] *Department of Biology, College of Science, Imam Abdulrahman Bin Faisal University, Dammam, Saudi Arabia*

[4] *Institute for Research and Medical Consultations, Imam Abdulrahman Bin Faisal University, Dammam, Saudi Arabia*

Abstract: This chapter covers the beneficial effect of curcumin, a biphenolic active compound of turmeric in diabetes and hypertension. Curcumin as a dietary component plays an important role in diabetes and hypertension inhibition as well as to mediate its anti-inflammatory effect by regulating redox status, transcription factors, fatty acids composition and various enzymatic activities. The active involvement of curcumin in the activation of activating peroxisome proliferator-activated receptor γ while the reduction in thiobarbituric acid reactive substances and succinate dehydrogenase is well known and correspondingly the disregulated adiokine which are involved in insulin resistance and development of Type 2 diabetes may be recovered by curcumin. The reduction in insulin resistance is induced by curcumin *via* activation of various transcription factors such as lipoprotein lipase, NF-E2-related factor 2, and liver enzymes involved in metabolic processes. Consequently, the molecular interaction of curcumin with adiponectin and signal transduction in various metabolic processes hinder insulin resistance, diabetes acceleration factors and other inflammatory symptoms linked with diabetes and hypertension.

Keywords: Adipokines, Curcumin, Diabetes, Hypertension, Inflammation.

INTRODUCTION

Curcumin treatment reduces blood glucose levels in diabetes patients by regulating antioxidant levels in pancreatic β-cells and by initiating peroxisome

* **Corresponding author Ebtesam A Al-Suhaimi:** Department of Biology, College of Science, Imam Abdulrahman Bin Faisal University (IAU), Dammam, Saudi Arabia; Institute for Research and Medical Consultations (IRMC), Imam Abdulrahman Bin Faisal University (IAU), Dammam, Saudi Arabia; Tel: +966133337007; E-mail: ealsuhaimi@iau.edu.sa

proliferator-actuated receptor γ (PPARγ) [1]. It additionally improved obesity related diabetes by diminishing macrophage penetration into white adipose tissue, hindering the depletion of κB (NFκB)-related markers of hepatic inflammation and increase adiponectin expression in high fat diet-induced obese and leptin-deficient ob/ob male C57BL/6J mice [2]. Moreover, curcumin is also reported to prevent diabetes-incited diminishes cancer prevention, increases in interleukin-1β (IL-1β), vascular endothelial advancement factor (VEGF), and NFκB, and covering of blood glucose levels through improved PPAR-γ ligand-confining activity in type II diabetic KK-Ay mice [3]. Curcumin hindered hyperlipidemia by stifling the serum and liver cholesterol [4]. In addition, curcumin pre-treatment guarantees against lindane-affected oxidative damage in rat's livers through the amplification of the enzymatic antioxidants [5]. This chapter aimed to provide the detailed underlying mechanisms of the multifactorial role of curcumin in the prevention and treatment of diabetes and hypertension (Table **1**).

Curcumin as a Drug of Choice for Diabetes

Scientific evidence has increased the impressive consideration of natural dietary products for the anticipation and diabetes and its associated diseases [3]. The active involvement of curcumin in diabetes treatment has been reported in traditional medicine (Fig. **1**). It is isolated as an active compound from the roots of *Curcuma longa*, which consists of curcuminoids such as curcumin, demethoxycurcumin, and bisdemethoxycurcumin [6]. Curcumin can manage the immune system positively, bringing about a significant impact on diabetes [7].

Curcumins' Antioxidant and Anti-Inflammatory Effect

Curcumin regulate a number of key proteins to facilitate its antioxidant effects. Initially, curcumin regulate redox status by modulating Ca^{2+} levels and protein kinase C (PKC) activity [8]. Furthermore, it inhibits ROS production by a blockage in apoptotic changes [9, 10]. Additionally, curcumin activates enzymatic antioxidants in Wistar-NIN rats [11]. Inflammation is a major cause of diabetes. It has been shown that curcumin restores membrane stiffening and reduces the release of pro-inflammatory factors, such as monocyte chemotactic protein-1 (MCP-1) from immune and endothelial cells [12, 13]. Curcumin also inhibits ILs, MCP-1, and tumor necrosis factor-α (TNF-α) in U937 monocytes. Similar effects were observed in diabetic mice by modulating TNF-α, IL-6, glucose, and glycated hemoglobin [13]. Curcumin inhibited the expression of acetylated CBP/p300 and p300, as well as NFκB, in human monocyte (THP-1) cells [14]. Furthermore, cytokine production was increased by high glucose levels *via* epigenetic changes, which regulate HAT and HDAC activity. Dietary curcumin inhibited both HATs and HDACs, thus contributing to epigenetic modifications for diabetes control [15].

Curcumin inhibited the degradation of IκBα and activation of NFκB, reduced macrophage infiltration, and down-regulated MCP-1, intracellular adhesion molecule-1 (ICAM-1) [16]. In insulin-resistant ob/ob mice with steatosis, curcumin improved peripheral insulin resistance by inhibiting NFκB/RelA DNA-binding activity, decreasing mRNA levels of IL-6 and TNF-α, and enhancing the production of IL-4 in adipose tissue macrophages and hepatic iNOS-producing dendritic cells [17]. Dietary curcumin decreased macrophage infiltration in white adipose tissue and hepatic NFκB activity, and ameliorated abnormal metabolic effects by increasing the production of adipose tissue adiponectin in high-fat diet-induced obesity and leptin-deficient ob/ob mice [18]. The potential role of curcumin in diabetes and hypertension-related diseases are discussed below.

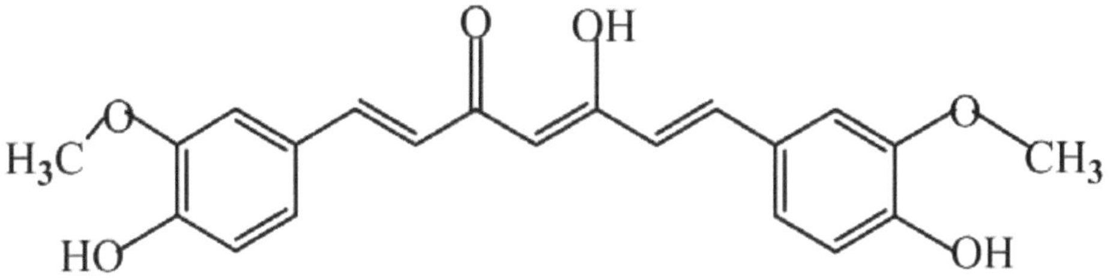

Fig. (1). Structure of Curcumin.

Curcumin Improves Adipose Tissue Dysfunction

Adipose tissue controls whole-body glucose homeostasis. Dysregulation of adiponectin secretion may lead to the development of T2DM [19, 20]. It has been reported that curcumin enhanced the differentiation of human adipocytes and blocked the accumulation and activation of macrophages in adipose tissue by regulating the secretion of adiponectin [21, 22]. Curcumin also suppressed NFκB activation and MCP-1 release in 3T3-L1 adipocytes [23]. Moreover, it suppressed adipogenesis *via* activation of β-catenin signaling D1 [24]. Both c-myc and cyclin D1 are well known downstream target genes of β-catenin and have the potential to prevent adipogenesis [25, 26].

Curcumin Inhibits Diabetes-Associated Liver Diseases

Most of the time diabetes patients develop liver diseases [27]. It has been reported that 8 weeks of curcumin administration improved STZ-induced diabetes in rats by modulating creatine, albumin, and inorganic phosphorus. Curcumin is also beneficial in reducing MDA level in urine and plasma [28]. Furthermore, the hypolipidemic action of curcumin is mediated by activation of hepatic cholesterol-7β-hydroxylase in STZ-induced diabetic rats [29]. Oral curcumin feeding decreased cholesterol, triglycerides, total lipids, and low density lipoprotein-cholesterol (LDL-c) in sodium arsenite-induced liver disorders [30]. It has been reported that curcumin improved lipidemia through activation of PPARγ, a central player in adipogenesis [31]. Improvement of lipidemia is correlated with the normalization of enzyme activity associated with glucose metabolism and lipid peroxidation [22, 32 - 34].

AMP-activated protein kinase (AMPK) controls glucose levels by stimulating their uptake and suppressing hepatic gluconeogenesis. Enzymes such as G6Paseand PEPCK have been reported to regulate hepatic gluconeogenesis, because overexpression of G6Pase and PEPCK mediate the harmful effects of diet-induced insulin resistance and T2DM [35]. It has been reported that curcumin inhibits PEPCK and G6Pase activity in Hep3B human hepatomas and H4IIE rat hepatoma cells [36]. Curcumin also inhibited the differentiation of Hep3B and H4IIE cells by targeting downstream target AMPK [11, 37, 38]. Curcumin eliminated the stimulatory effects of leptin on HSCs by activating AMPK, leading to lipid accumulation [39]. Curcumin also down-regulates LOX-1 and Wnt, and stimulates the activity of receptor for advanced glycation endproducts (RAGE) and PPARγ, thereby inhibiting fat accumulation [40].

Curcumin administration prevents liver fat accumulation in high-fat diet (HFD) fed rats. Furthermore, curcumin mediates antilipolytic and anti-inflammatory properties and decreased plasma free fatty acid and TNFα levels [41, 42]. In a clinical trial, 63 acute coronary syndrome patients were feed with 45 mg/d curcumin for 60 days, which resulted in reduction of LDL cholesterol and total cholesterol levels [43].

Curcumin Improves Pancreatic Cells Dysfunction

There are clear evidences of pancreatic β-cell functions and hyperglycemia improvement by curcumin treatment. Curcumin induced electrical pulses by volume-regulated anion channel activation in rat pancreatic β-cells [44]. Curcumin activated anion channels and decreased β -cell volume, reflecting a loss of Cl- and water, suggesting that Cl- flux plays a major role in regulating β- cell function. In addition to stimulation of β-cell function, curcumin was reported to induce heme oxygenase-1 expression, which has cytoprotective effects in mouse pancreatic β-cells [45]. These effects were mediated through the activation of Nrf2. Further work demonstrated that curcumin treatment enhanced islet recovery in various experimental studies [46].

Curcumin Prevents Neuropathy

Diabetic neuropathy is a nerve disorder caused by T2DM. Diabetes can induce microvascular injury, increase advanced glycation endproducts (AGE), and activate PKC, leading to diabetic neuropathy [47]. Studies have shown that curcumin treatment efficiently improves neuropathic disorders. Curcumin elevated reduced glutathione levels, modulated lipid peroxidation, and enhanced antioxidant enzymes activity, further inhibiting the development of diabetic cataracts in STZinduced diabetic rats [48, 49]. Curcumin has been shown to regulate osmotic stress by polyol pathway [50]. Curcumin also prevented lens protein aggregation and loss of solubilization induced by hyperglycemia.

Curcumin influenced apoptosis in human retinal endothelial cells (HREC) by blocking VEGF and PKC-2 activation [51]. Curcumin inhibited stromal-derived factor-1 (SDF-1) activation of HRECs by supressing Ca^{2+} influx, followed by reduction of PI3K/Akt signaling [52]. In contrast, curcumin mediated antioxidant effects by modulating 8-OHdG, glutathione, and SOD/catalase under certain conditions [53]. Curcumin also inhibited nucleotide excision repair enzyme activation in the retina of STZ-induced diabetic rats [51, 54, 55]. Curcumin has also improved diabetes associated cognitive defects [55]. Curcumin attenuated cholinergic dysfunction by modulating the activation of dopamine (D1, D2) receptors, cAMP response element binding protein (CREB), GLUT3, phospholipase C, and the insulin receptor [56, 57]. These changes may occur due to a curcumin-induced reduction in glutamate-mediated excitotoxicity in diabetic rats [58]. Curcumin reduced single-minded 2 (Sim2), which is associated with hyperglycemia-induced neuronal injury and impaired learning capacity [59]. Curcumin also blocked amyloid oligomers and improved cognitive deficits through phosphorylation and degradation of the insulin receptor substrate in cultured hippocampal neurons [60]. Furthermore, curcumin significantly inhibited allodynia and hyperalgesia in diabetic mice [61] as well in rats [62, 63] with or without gliclazide, an antidiabetic drug by its various neuroprotective effects [64, 65].

Curcumin Prevents Nephropathy

Curcumin ameliorated macrophage infiltration through blocking NFκB and other inflammatory markers in STZ-induced diabetic nephropathy [66]. Further, it altered posttranslational modifications of histone H3, heat-shock protein-27, and p38 MAP kinase in STZ-induced type I diabetic nephropathy [67]. In line with these data, curcumin also inhibited p300 in diabetic kidneys [68]. It played a prominent role in activating the p38 MAP kinase-HSP25 pathway in mouse podocytes; however, treatment did not significantly reduce albumin level in STZ model of diabetes [69]. These effects may be mediated by activation of AMPK [70], which down-regulates VEGF and the VEGF receptor [71], reduces PKC activity [72], and suppresses sterol regulatory element-binding protein (SREBP)

[70]. Clinical trials showed that curcumin reduces TGF-α, IL-8, and urinary protein levels in diabetic neuropathy patients [73].

Curcumin in Diabetic Vascular Diseases

Curcumin treatment decreased endothelial nitric oxide synthase (eNOS) and iNOS levels, thereby inhibiting DNA oxidation and protein damage in the heart in STZ-induced diabetic rats [74]. Curcumin also prevented NFκB and AP-1 mediated alterations in NOS and oxidative stress. Microvascular endothelial cells showed elevated ET- 1 levels after exposure to curcumin. Besides, curcumin prevented diabetic vascular abnormalities by blocking diabetes-induced upregulation of p300 [75].

Curcumin General Role in Diabetes Related Complications

Several studies have demonstrated that curcumin prevents diabetes-induced musculoskeletal diseases (Fig. **2**). Studies indicated that diabetes-stimulated bone resorption was suppressed by curcumin treatment through the reduction of tartrate-resistant acid phosphatase and cathepsin K, followed by inhibition of c-fos and c-jun expression [76]. Curcumin improved the expression of GLUT4 through the phospholipase C-PI3K pathway, and improved insulin resistance in muscle tissue through the liver kinase B1 (LKB1)-AMPK pathway, resulting in increased glucose uptake in skeletal muscle [77, 78]. Curcumin treatment also decreased insulin receptor substrate-1 (IRS-1) phosphorylation on Ser307 and activated Akt phosphorylation in skeletal muscles [79]. Additionally, vitamin D3 and curcumin suppressed Akt, CREB, the insulin receptor, 2-adrenoceptor, and malate dehydrogenase activity [80].

Curcumin can prevent diabetes-induced erectile dysfunction by enhancing cGMP levels, HO-1, eNOS, intracavernosal pressure (ICP), neuronal NOS (nNOS), and Nrf2, while concomitantly reducing p38 MAP kinase, NF κB, and iNOS levels [81]. Curcumin ameliorated STZ-induced testicular damage and apoptotic germ cell death through its antioxidant effects [82]. A study conducted on diabetic gastroparesis rats revealed that feeding of dietary curcumin for 42 days significantly improved the rate of gastric emptying, decreased MDA levels, and increased SOD activity. This effect involves an antioxidant-based mechanism, resulting in elevated expression of SCF/c-kit [83 - 85].

HYPERTENSION

The use of curcumin to treat and prevent hypertension has been well studied. Curcumin regulate a number of molecular targets *in-vitro* and *in-vivo*, consequently eradicate the harmful effects of hypertension [86, 87].

Therapeutic Role of Curcumin in Hypertension

Curcumin Improves the Function of the Aorta

Hypertension is accompanied by functional and morphological changes in the vascular wall. Curcumin was administered for six weeks in NG-nitro-L-arginine methyl ester (L-NAME)-induced hypertensive rats. Hypertension was associated with inhibition of NO synthases and decreased NO production [87, 88]. Curcumin administration reversed L-NAME-induced hypertension in rats and increased NO production [87]. Further, curcumin decreases iNOS expression and stimulated eNOS [87]. In another study, curcumin was tested in combination with piperine in L-NAME-induced hypertension [89]. L-NAME increased hypertension by increasing aortic media thickness and cross-sectional area, accompanied by an increased proportion of Mallory's phosphotungstic acid hematoxylin (PTAH)-positive myofibrils, and decrease in elastin, actin, and collagen [89]. Piperine decreased the myofibril content and slightly raised the proportion of actin, whereas curcumin prevented elevated elastin levels [90]. The combined effect of both compounds on vessel morphology was the same as curcumin alone. Single administration of curcumin was more effective in preventing abnormal changes in blood vessel morphology accompanying hypertensive disease [89].

Curcumin Prevents Heart Failure

A study conducted in two different models of heart failure, hypertension, and myocardial infarction, demonstrated that curcumin prevented deterioration of systolic function and had no effect on systemic hemodynamics. Curcumin efficiently decreased left ventricular wall thickness, as well as the diameter of myocytes in both models. Inhibition of cardiomyocyte hypertrophy with curcumin was accompanied by reduced gene expression of brain natriuretic peptide [91]. Although perivascular fibrosis was significantly reduced by curcumin treatment, the effect was minimal. In rat myocytes that underwent myocardial infarction, curcumin decreased the wall thickness and diameter to nearly the same level as sham-operated rats. Curcumin also inhibited hypertension-induced acetylation of GATA4 and formation of p300/GATA4 complexes in salt-sensitive Dahl rats [92].

Curcumin has the ability to inhibit the p300-mediated acetylation of p53 *in vitro* and *in vivo*. Curcumin disrupts the conformation of the p53 required for its serine phosphorylation [93]. Recently, it has been reported that sustained hypertension results in an accumulation of p53, which blocks hypoxia-inducible factor-1 (HIF-1) activity. This blockage leads to cardiac angiogenesis impairment and heart failure [94]. Curcumin is reported to block transcriptional activation of NFκB

[95]. Importantly, inhibition of NFκB is an important strategy to control cardiomyocyte hypertrophy [96]. It has been reported that curcumin protects against isoproterenol-induced myocardial necrosis in rats and that this protective effect is mediated by its antioxidant action [97]. In the future, the multiple actions of curcumin and its ability to target nuclear signaling pathways in cardiomyocytes will provide a novel therapeutic strategy against heart failure.

Curcumin in Idiopathic Pulmonary Arterial Hypertension

The drugs available to treat IPAH are few, expensive, and require combination therapy. They are also associated with various adverse effects. Curcumin could be a possible therapeutic solution for IPAH. Curcumin suppresses the NFκB pathway and inflammatory cytokines, including IL-1β, IL-6, and IL-8. Curcumin also regulates cyclooxygenase-2 (COX-2) production and TNF-α, consequently improving IPAH [98]. In addition, curcumin modulates iNOS, phospholipase A2 (PLA2), and 5-LOX in pulmonary arteries [99 - 101]. However, curcumin is a double edge sword for the treatment of IPAH, because it inhibits the inflammatory process and controls the arterial remodeling. Curcumin also inhibits NFκB gene products, followed by suppression of cell proliferation and survival genes [98]. iNOS modulation by curcumin regulates cGMP activity, promoting vasodilation and inhibiting proliferation [101]. COX-2, PLA2, and 5-LOX modulation regulates the arachidonic acid pathway, and consequently prostacyclin production, which promotes vasodilation and inhibits proliferation [100, 101]. Curcumin is a low cost and well-tolerated drug with minimum toxicity. Thus, daily intake could be beneficial.

Curcumin Regulate Adipokines

Curcumin down regulates the adipokines, resistin and leptin, while up-regulates adiponectin and related proteins. Curcumins communication with numerous signal transduction routs reverse insulin resistance, hyperglycaemia, hyperlipidaemia [11]. Curcumin has been displayed to reveal pleiotropic properties by modulating different signaling molecules, such as transcription factors, adipokines, and cytokines. Dysregulation of adipokines, including adiponectin, leptin, resistin, and visfatin, are involved in the development of insulin resistance and Type 2 diabetes [11, 102].

High fructose diet (HFD) induced metabolic syndrome (MetS) while curcumin in presence of HFD, improved significant glucose and lipid metabolism estimations, and also regulates oxidative stress and inflammation biomarker. Curcumin is possibly helpful in curing MetS by its reducing oxidation stress and inflammation flows [103].

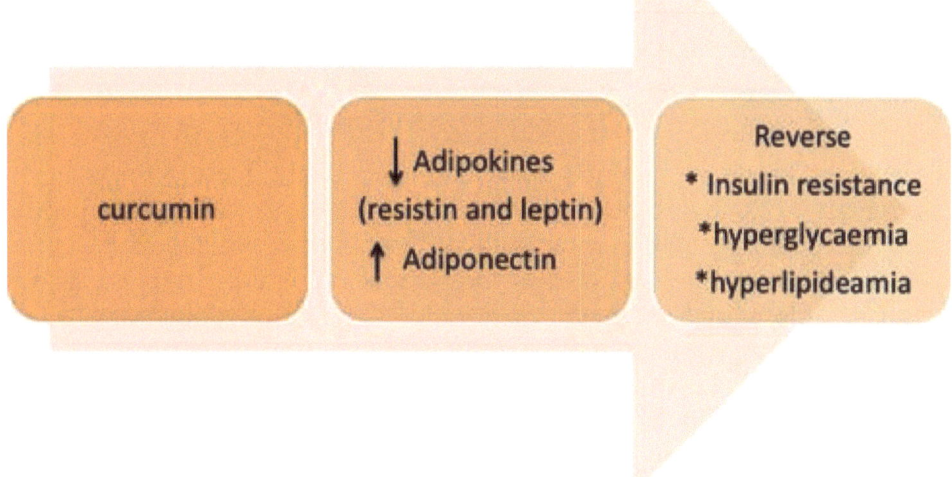

Fig. (2). Curcumin reverses insulin resistance, hyperglycemia and hyperlipidemia, by downregulating adipokines (resistin and leptin) and upregulating adiponectin.

A recent study on the variations in serum concentrations of cancer Antigen 125 (CA125), leptin, resistin, homocysteine, and total antioxidant capacity in an experimental rat model of endometriosis and explored the influence of curcumin treatment on these adipokines and parameters. They found that curcumin can avoid the growth of endometriosis without significant changes in the studied factors [104].

NANOCURCUMIN AGAINST DIABETES

Previous phrmacological studies have shown intracellular delivery with high efficacy and therapeutic effects for nanoparticles due to their size and surface characteristics. Recently, nanoformulations of curcumin such as nanoparticles, liposomes, micelles, phospholipids, and curcumin-encapsulated polymer nanoparticles are practiced to overcome for low bioavailability as well as for advance therapeutic effect [25]. Previous studies have shown that nanocurcumin has improved antidiabetic effects as compared to normal curcumin formulations. In a double blind randomized clinical trials, nanocurcumin (nano-micelle 80 mg/day) treatment for 3 months decreased HbA1C, FBG, TG, and BMI followed by partially decrease in serum LDL-C in type-2 diabetes [105]. Nanocurcumin has the ability to induce hypoglycemia, and increases the gene expression of insulin and insulin receptor in STZ-induced diabetic rats [106]. Nanocurcumin 10 or 50 mg/kg treatment reduced glucose level, decreased islet or β cell death in non-fasted rats pretreated with STZ. A big difference has been noted in nano and normal curcumin in decreasing the inflammatory cytokines and 8-oxo-2'-deoxyguanosine in pancreas that correlated well with minimal histiocytic infiltration. Also, no harmful effect has been noted with treatment of nCUR (25-100 mg/kg) for 28 days in normal rodents [107].

CONCLUSION

Based on recent research curcumin has shown beneficial effects in the prevention and treatment of diabetes and hypertension and their associated disorders. Regarding diabetes, curcumin could favorably affect hyperglycemia. Curcumin also prevented detrimental worst effects of diabetes. Clinical trials of curcumin are only available in diabetic nephropathy, microangiopathy, and retinopathy to date. The therapeutic applications of curcumin can be further confirmed in large scale human studies. To fully address these concerns, more large-scale human studies are needed. In the case of hypertension, curcumin has been shown to be effective in remodeling the aorta, suppressing p300 histone acetyltransferase level, and preventing cardiac failure and IPAH.

Conversely, few studies have shown that curcumin (200 mg/kg. b. wt.) treatment for 14 days has mild effect on blood glucose and insulin levels in STZ-induced diabetic rats [108]. In line with this, curcumin (200 mg/kg b. wt.) has no significant effect on blood glucose in STZ diabetic rats [33]. This is not the matter of curcumin, but it seems the subject of different models, dose and/or rout of dosage of curcumin or nano-curcumin. This can be achieved by nanoformultions, and other sustained release studies. Once the desired results achieved, curcumin will be a drug of choice for the treatment of diabetes and hypertension in the near future.

CONSENT FOR PUBLICATION

Not applicable.

CONFLICT OF INTEREST

There is no conflict of interest declared.

ACKNOWLEDGEMENT

Declared none.

REFERENCES

[1]   Aldebasi YH, Aly SM, Rahmani AH. Therapeutic implications of curcumin in the prevention of diabetic retinopathy *via* modulation of anti-oxidant activity and genetic pathways. Int J Physiol Pathophysiol Pharmacol 2013; 5(4): 194-202.
[PMID: 24379904]

[2]   Weisberg SP, Leibel R, Tortoriello DV. Dietary curcumin significantly improves obesity-associated inflammation and diabetes in mouse models of diabesity. Endocrinology 2008; 149(7): 3549-58.
[http://dx.doi.org/10.1210/en.2008-0262] [PMID: 18403477]

[3]   Shehzad A, Lee J, Lee YS. Curcumin in various cancers. Biofactors 2013; 39(1): 56-68.
[http://dx.doi.org/10.1002/biof.1068] [PMID: 23303705]

[4]   Pari L, Murugan P. Antihyperlipidemic effect of curcumin and tetrahydrocurcumin in experimental type 2 diabetic rats. Ren Fail 2007; 29(7): 881-9.
[http://dx.doi.org/10.1080/08860220701540326] [PMID: 17994458]

[5]   Palipoch S, Punsawad C, Koomhin P, Suwannalert P. Hepatoprotective effect of curcumin and alpha-tocopherol against cisplatin-induced oxidative stress. BMC Complement Altern Med 2014; 14: 111.
[http://dx.doi.org/10.1186/1472-6882-14-111] [PMID: 24674233]

[6]   Shehzad A, Lee YS. Molecular mechanisms of curcumin action: signal transduction. Biofactors 2013; 39(1): 27-36.
[http://dx.doi.org/10.1002/biof.1065] [PMID: 23303697]

[7]   Jagetia GC, Aggarwal BB. "Spicing up" of the immune system by curcumin. J Clin Immunol 2007; 27(1): 19-35.
[http://dx.doi.org/10.1007/s10875-006-9066-7] [PMID: 17211725]

[8]   Shehzad A, Wahid F, Lee YS. Curcumin in cancer chemoprevention: molecular targets, pharmacokinetics, bioavailability, and clinical trials. Arch Pharm (Weinheim) 2010; 343(9): 489-99.
[http://dx.doi.org/10.1002/ardp.200900319] [PMID: 20726007]

[9]   Shehzad A, Khan S, Shehzad O, Lee YS. Curcumin therapeutic promises and bioavailability in colorectal cancer. Drugs Today (Barc) 2010; 46(7): 523-32.
[http://dx.doi.org/10.1358/dot.2010.46.7.1509560] [PMID: 20683505]

[10]   Chan WH, Wu HJ, Hsuuw YD. Curcumin inhibits ROS formation and apoptosis in methylglyoxal-treated human hepatoma G2 cells. Ann N Y Acad Sci 2005; 1042: 372-8.
[http://dx.doi.org/10.1196/annals.1338.057] [PMID: 15965083]

[11]   Shehzad A, Ha T, Subhan F, Lee YS. New mechanisms and the anti-inflammatory role of curcumin in obesity and obesity-related metabolic diseases. Eur J Nutr 2011; 50(3): 151-61.
[http://dx.doi.org/10.1007/s00394-011-0188-1] [PMID: 21442412]

[12]   Margina D, Gradinaru D, Manda G, Neagoe I, Ilie M. Membranar effects exerted *in vitro* by polyphenols - quercetin, epigallocatechin gallate and curcumin - on HUVEC and Jurkat cells, relevant for diabetes mellitus. Food Chem Toxicol 2013; 61: 86-93.
[http://dx.doi.org/10.1016/j.fct.2013.02.046] [PMID: 23466460]

[13]   Jain SK, Rains J, Croad J, Larson B, Jones K. Curcumin supplementation lowers TNF-α, IL-6, IL-8, and MCP-1 secretion in high glucose-treated cultured monocytes and blood levels of TNF-α, IL-6, MCP-1, glucose, and glycosylated hemoglobin in diabetic rats. Antioxid Redox Signal 2009; 11(2): 241-9.
[http://dx.doi.org/10.1089/ars.2008.2140] [PMID: 18976114]

[14]   Yun JM, Jialal I, Devaraj S. Epigenetic regulation of high glucose-induced proinflammatory cytokine production in monocytes by curcumin. J Nutr Biochem 2011; 22(5): 450-8.
[http://dx.doi.org/10.1016/j.jnutbio.2010.03.014] [PMID: 20655188]

[15]   Shehzad A, Khan S, Sup Lee Y. Curcumin molecular targets in obesity and obesity-related cancers. Future Oncol 2012; 8(2): 179-90.
[http://dx.doi.org/10.2217/fon.11.145] [PMID: 22335582]

[16]   Soetikno V, Sari FR, Veeraveedu PT, *et al.* Curcumin ameliorates macrophage infiltration by inhibiting NF-κB activation and proinflammatory cytokines in streptozotocin induced-diabetic nephropathy. Nutr Metab (Lond) 2011; 8(1): 35.
[http://dx.doi.org/10.1186/1743-7075-8-35] [PMID: 21663638]

[17]   Yekollu SK, Thomas R, O'Sullivan B. Targeting curcusomes to inflammatory dendritic cells inhibits NF-κB and improves insulin resistance in obese mice. Diabetes 2011; 60(11): 2928-38.
[http://dx.doi.org/10.2337/db11-0275] [PMID: 21885868]

[18]   Shehzad A, Shahzad R, Lee YS. Curcumin: A potent modulator of multiple enzymes in multiple cancers.The Enzymes. 149-74.

[19]   Majithiya JB, Balaraman R. Time-dependent changes in antioxidant enzymes and vascular reactivity of aorta in streptozotocin-induced diabetic rats treated with curcumin. J Cardiovasc Pharmacol 2005; 46(5): 697-705.
[http://dx.doi.org/10.1097/01.fjc.0000183720.85014.24] [PMID: 16220078]

[20]   Shehzad A, Lee J, Huh TL, Lee YS. Curcumin induces apoptosis in human colorectal carcinoma (HCT-15) cells by regulating expression of Prp4 and p53. Mol Cells 2013; 35(6): 526-32.
[http://dx.doi.org/10.1007/s10059-013-0038-5] [PMID: 23686430]

[21]   Pérez-Torres I, Ruiz-Ramírez A, Baños G, El-Hafidi M. Hibiscus sabdariffa Linnaeus (Malvaceae), curcumin and resveratrol as alternative medicinal agents against metabolic syndrome. Cardiovasc Hematol Agents Med Chem 2013; 11(1): 25-37.
[http://dx.doi.org/10.2174/1871525711311010006] [PMID: 22721439]

[22]   Shehzad A, Rehman G, Lee YS. Curcumin in inflammatory diseases. Biofactors 2013; 39(1): 69-77.
[http://dx.doi.org/10.1002/biof.1066] [PMID: 23281076]

[23]   Shehzad A, Park JW, Lee J, Lee YS. Curcumin induces radiosensitivity of *in vitro* and *in vivo* cancer models by modulating pre-mRNA processing factor 4 (Prp4). Chem Biol Interact 2013; 206(2): 394-402.
[http://dx.doi.org/10.1016/j.cbi.2013.10.007] [PMID: 24144778]

[24]   Ahn J, Lee H, Kim S, Ha T. Curcumin-induced suppression of adipogenic differentiation is accompanied by activation of Wnt/β-catenin signaling. Am J Physiol Cell Physiol 2010; 298(6): C1510-6.
[http://dx.doi.org/10.1152/ajpcell.00369.2009] [PMID: 20357182]

[25]   Shehzad A, Ul-Islam M, Wahid F, Lee YS. Multifunctional polymeric nanocurcumin for cancer therapy. J Nanosci Nanotechnol 2014; 14(1): 803-14.
[http://dx.doi.org/10.1166/jnn.2014.9103] [PMID: 24730299]

[26]   Shehzad A, Rehmat S, Islam SU, Ahmad R, Al-Suhaimi EA. Ether inhibits NF-κB and COX-2 and activates IκBα expressions in CCl4-induced hepatic fibrosis BMC Complementary and Alternative Medicine 2020. BCAM D-19-01076

[27]   Prentki M, Madiraju SR. Glycerolipid metabolism and signaling in health and disease. Endocr Rev 2008; 29(6): 647-76.
[http://dx.doi.org/10.1210/er.2008-0007] [PMID: 18606873]

[28]   Babu PS, Srinivasan K. Influence of dietary curcumin and cholesterol on the progression of experimentally induced diabetes in albino rat. Mol Cell Biochem 1995; 152(1): 13-21.
[PMID: 8609907]

[29]   Babu PS, Srinivasan K. Hypolipidemic action of curcumin, the active principle of turmeric (*Curcuma longa*) in streptozotocin induced diabetic rats. Mol Cell Biochem 1997; 166(1-2): 169-75.
[http://dx.doi.org/10.1023/A:1006819605211] [PMID: 9046034]

[30]   Yousef MI, El-Demerdash FM, Radwan FM. Sodium arsenite induced biochemical perturbations in rats: ameliorating effect of curcumin. Food Chem Toxicol 2008; 46(11): 3506-11.
[http://dx.doi.org/10.1016/j.fct.2008.08.031] [PMID: 18809455]

[31]   Nishiyama T, Mae T, Kishida H, *et al.* Curcuminoids and sesquiterpenoids in turmeric (*Curcuma longa* L.) suppress an increase in blood glucose level in type 2 diabetic KK-Ay mice. J Agric Food Chem 2005; 53(4): 959-63.
[http://dx.doi.org/10.1021/jf0483873] [PMID: 15713005]

[32]   Seo KI, Choi MS, Jung UJ, *et al.* Effect of curcumin supplementation on blood glucose, plasma insulin, and glucose homeostasis related enzyme activities in diabetic db/db mice. Mol Nutr Food Res 2008; 52(9): 995-1004.
[http://dx.doi.org/10.1002/mnfr.200700184] [PMID: 18398869]

[33]   Shehzad A, Iqbal W, Shehzad O, Lee YS. Adiponectin: regulation of its production and its role in human diseases. Hormones (Athens) 2012; 11(1): 8-20.
[http://dx.doi.org/10.1007/BF03401534] [PMID: 22450341]

[34]   Gutierres VO, Pinheiro CM, Assis RP, Vendramini RC, Pepato MT, Brunetti IL. Curcumin-supplemented yoghurt improves physiological and biochemical markers of experimental diabetes. Br J Nutr 2012; 108(3): 440-8.
[http://dx.doi.org/10.1017/S0007114511005769] [PMID: 22067670]

[35]   Franckhauser S, Muñoz S, Elias I, Ferre T, Bosch F. Adipose overexpression of phosphoenolpyruvate carboxykinase leads to high susceptibility to diet-induced insulin resistance and obesity. Diabetes 2006; 55(2): 273-80.
[http://dx.doi.org/10.2337/diabetes.55.02.06.db05-0482] [PMID: 16443757]

[36]   Kim T, Davis J, Zhang AJ, He X, Mathews ST. Curcumin activates AMPK and suppresses gluconeogenic gene expression in hepatoma cells. Biochem Biophys Res Commun 2009; 388(2): 377-82.
[http://dx.doi.org/10.1016/j.bbrc.2009.08.018] [PMID: 19665995]

[37]   Fujiwara H, Hosokawa M, Zhou X, *et al.* Curcumin inhibits glucose production in isolated mice hepatocytes. Diabetes Res Clin Pract 2008; 80(2): 185-91.
[http://dx.doi.org/10.1016/j.diabres.2007.12.004] [PMID: 18221818]

[38]   Shehzad A, Islam Ul. Prostaglandin E2 reverses curcumin-induced inhibition of survival signal pathways in human colorectal carcinoma (HCT-15) cell lines Mol Cells 2014; b37(12): 899-906.

[39]   Tang Y, Chen A. Curcumin protects hepatic stellate cells against leptin-induced activation *in vitro* by accumulating intracellular lipids. Endocrinology 2010; 151(9): 4168-77.
[http://dx.doi.org/10.1210/en.2010-0191] [PMID: 20660066]

[40]   Aggarwal BB. Targeting inflammation-induced obesity and metabolic diseases by curcumin and other nutraceuticals. Annu Rev Nutr 2010; 30: 173-99.
[http://dx.doi.org/10.1146/annurev.nutr.012809.104755] [PMID: 20420526]

[41]   Xie XY, Kong PR, Wu JF, Li Y, Li YX. Curcumin attenuates lipolysis stimulated by tumor necrosis factor-α or isoproterenol in 3T3-L1 adipocytes. Phytomedicine 2012; 20(1): 3-8.
[http://dx.doi.org/10.1016/j.phymed.2012.09.003] [PMID: 23083815]

[42]   Öner-İyidoğan Y, Koçak H, Seyidhanoğlu M, *et al.* Curcumin prevents liver fat accumulation and serum fetuin-A increase in rats fed a high-fat diet. J Physiol Biochem 2013; 69(4): 677-86.
[http://dx.doi.org/10.1007/s13105-013-0244-9] [PMID: 23430567]

[43]   Alwi I, Santoso T, Suyono S, *et al.* The effect of curcumin on lipid level in patients with acute coronary syndrome. Acta Med Indones 2008; 40(4): 201-10.
[PMID: 19151449]

[44]   Best L, Elliott AC, Brown PD. Curcumin induces electrical activity in rat pancreatic beta-cells by activating the volume-regulated anion channel. Biochem Pharmacol 2007; 73(11): 1768-75.
[http://dx.doi.org/10.1016/j.bcp.2007.02.006] [PMID: 17382910]

[45]   Pugazhenthi S, Akhov L, Selvaraj G, Wang M, Alam J. Regulation of heme oxygenase-1 expression by demethoxy curcuminoids through Nrf2 by a PI3-kinase/Akt-mediated pathway in mouse beta-cells. Am J Physiol Endocrinol Metab 2007; 293(3): E645-55.
[http://dx.doi.org/10.1152/ajpendo.00111.2007] [PMID: 17535857]

[46]   Kanitkar M, Bhonde RR. Curcumin treatment enhances islet recovery by induction of heat shock response proteins, Hsp70 and heme oxygenase-1, during cryopreservation. Life Sci 2008; 82(3-4):

182-9.
[http://dx.doi.org/10.1016/j.lfs.2007.10.026] [PMID: 18093618]

[47]   Joshi RP, Negi G, Kumar A, *et al.* SNEDDS curcumin formulation leads to enhanced protection from pain and functional deficits associated with diabetic neuropathy: an insight into its mechanism for neuroprotection. Nanomedicine (Lond) 2013; 9(6): 776-85.
[http://dx.doi.org/10.1016/j.nano.2013.01.001] [PMID: 23347896]

[48]   Kumar PA, Suryanarayana P, Reddy PY, Reddy GB. Modulation of α-crystallin chaperone activity in diabetic rat lens by curcumin. Mol Vis 2005; 11: 561-8.
[PMID: 16088325]

[49]   Kumar PA, Haseeb A, Suryanarayana P, Ehtesham NZ, Reddy GB. Elevated expression of alphaA- and alphaB-crystallins in streptozotocin-induced diabetic rat. Arch Biochem Biophys 2005; 444(2): 77-83.
[http://dx.doi.org/10.1016/j.abb.2005.09.021] [PMID: 16309625]

[50]   Suryanarayana P, Saraswat M, Mrudula T, Krishna TP, Krishnaswamy K, Reddy GB. Curcumin and mturmeric delay streptozotocin-induced diabetic cataract in rats Invest Ophthalmol Vis Sci 2005; m46(6): 9-2092.

[51]   Premanand C, Rema M, Sameer MZ, Sujatha M, Balasubramanyam M. Effect of curcumin on proliferation of human retinal endothelial cells under *in vitro* conditions. Invest Ophthalmol Vis Sci 2006; 47(5): 2179-84.
[http://dx.doi.org/10.1167/iovs.05-0580] [PMID: 16639030]

[52]   Sameermahmood Z, Balasubramanyam M, Saravanan T, Rema M. Curcumin modulates SDF-1α/CXCR4-induced migration of human retinal endothelial cells (HRECs). Invest Ophthalmol Vis Sci 2008; 49(8): 3305-11.
[http://dx.doi.org/10.1167/iovs.07-0456] [PMID: 18660423]

[53]   Gupta SK, Kumar B, Nag TC, *et al.* Curcumin prevents experimental diabetic retinopathy in rats through its hypoglycemic, antioxidant, and anti-inflammatory mechanisms. J Ocul Pharmacol Ther 2011; 27(2): 123-30.
[http://dx.doi.org/10.1089/jop.2010.0123] [PMID: 21314438]

[54]   Shehzad A, Qureshi M, Anwar MN, Lee YS. Multifunctional curcumin mediate multitherapeutic effects. J Food Sci 2017; 82(9): 2006-15.
[http://dx.doi.org/10.1111/1750-3841.13793] [PMID: 28771714]

[55]   Kuhad A, Chopra K. Curcumin attenuates diabetic encephalopathy in rats: behavioral and biochemical evidences. Eur J Pharmacol 2007; 576(1-3): 34-42.
[http://dx.doi.org/10.1016/j.ejphar.2007.08.001] [PMID: 17822693]

[56]   Kumar TP, Antony S, Gireesh G, George N, Paulose CS. Curcumin modulates dopaminergic receptor, CREB and phospholipase C gene expression in the cerebral cortex and cerebellum of streptozotocin induced diabetic rats. J Biomed Sci 2010; 17: 43.
[http://dx.doi.org/10.1186/1423-0127-17-43] [PMID: 20513244]

[57]   Peeyush Kumar T, Antony S, Soman S, Kuruvilla KP, George N, Paulose CS. Role of curcumin in the prevention of cholinergic mediated cortical dysfunctions in streptozotocin-induced diabetic rats mMol Cell Endocrinol 2011; 331(1): 1-10.

[58]   Jayanarayanan S, Smijin S, Peeyush KT, Anju TR, Paulose CS. NMDA and AMPA receptor mediated excitotoxicity in cerebral cortex of streptozotocin induced diabetic rat: ameliorating effects of curcumin. Chem Biol Interact 2013; 201(1-3): 39-48.
[http://dx.doi.org/10.1016/j.cbi.2012.11.024] [PMID: 23267840]

[59]   Wang X, Song Y, Chen L, *et al.* Contribution of single-minded 2 to hyperglycaemia-induced neurotoxicity. Neurotoxicology 2013; 35: 106-12.
[http://dx.doi.org/10.1016/j.neuro.2013.01.003] [PMID: 23333261]

[60]   Ma QL, Yang F, Rosario ER, *et al.* β-amyloid oligomers induce phosphorylation of tau and inactivation of insulin receptor substrate *via* c-Jun N-terminal kinase signaling: suppression by omega-3 fatty acids and curcumin. J Neurosci 2009; 29(28): 9078-89.
[http://dx.doi.org/10.1523/JNEUROSCI.1071-09.2009] [PMID: 19605645]

[61]   Sharma S, Kulkarni SK, Agrewala JN, Chopra K. Curcumin attenuates thermal hyperalgesia in a diabetic mouse model of neuropathic pain. Eur J Pharmacol 2006; 536(3): 256-61.
[http://dx.doi.org/10.1016/j.ejphar.2006.03.006] [PMID: 16584726]

[62]   Attia HN, Al-Rasheed NM, Al-Rasheed NM, Maklad YA, Ahmed AA, Kenawy SA. Protective effects of combined therapy of gliclazide with curcumin in experimental diabetic neuropathy in rats. Behav Pharmacol 2012; 23(2): 153-61.
[http://dx.doi.org/10.1097/FBP.0b013e3283512c00] [PMID: 22411174]

[63]   Li Y, Zhang Y, Liu DB, Liu HY, Hou WG, Dong YS. Curcumin attenuates diabetic neuropathic pain by downregulating TNF-α in a rat model. Int J Med Sci 2013; 10(4): 377-81.
[http://dx.doi.org/10.7150/ijms.5224] [PMID: 23471081]

[64]   Sharma S, Chopra K, Kulkarni SK. Effect of insulin and its combination with resveratrol or curcumin in attenuation of diabetic neuropathic pain: participation of nitric oxide and TNF-alpha. Phytother Res 2007; 21(3): 278-83.
[http://dx.doi.org/10.1002/ptr.2070] [PMID: 17199240]

[65]   Acar A, Akil E, Alp H, *et al.* Oxidative damage is ameliorated by curcumin treatment in brain and sciatic nerve of diabetic rats. Int J Neurosci 2012; 122(7): 367-72.
[http://dx.doi.org/10.3109/00207454.2012.657380] [PMID: 22248035]

[66]   Soetikno V, Sari FR, Veeraveedu PT, *et al.* Curcumin ameliorates macrophage infiltration by inhibiting NF-κB activation and proinflammatory cytokines in streptozotocin induced-diabetic nephropathy. Nutr Metab (Lond) 2011; 8(1): 35.
[http://dx.doi.org/10.1186/1743-7075-8-35] [PMID: 21663638]

[67]   Tikoo K, Meena RL, Kabra DG, Gaikwad AB. Change in post-translational modifications of histone H3, heat-shock protein-27 and MAP kinase p38 expression by curcumin in streptozotocin-induced type I diabetic nephropathy. Br J Pharmacol 2008; 153(6): 1225-31.
[http://dx.doi.org/10.1038/sj.bjp.0707666] [PMID: 18204486]

[68]   Chiu J, Khan ZA, Farhangkhoee H, Chakrabarti S. Curcumin prevents diabetes-associated abnormalities in the kidneys by inhibiting p300 and nuclear factor-kappaB. Nutrition 2009; 25(9): 964-72.
[http://dx.doi.org/10.1016/j.nut.2008.12.007] [PMID: 19268536]

[69]   Ma J, Phillips L, Wang Y, *et al.* Curcumin activates the p38MPAK-HSP25 pathway *in vitro* but fails to attenuate diabetic nephropathy in DBA2J mice despite urinary clearance documented by HPLC. BMC Complement Altern Med 2010; 10: 67.
[http://dx.doi.org/10.1186/1472-6882-10-67] [PMID: 21073732]

[70]   Soetikno V, Sari FR, Sukumaran V, *et al.* Curcumin decreases renal triglyceride accumulation through AMPK-SREBP signaling pathway in streptozotocin-induced type 1 diabetic rats. J Nutr Biochem 2013; 24(5): 796-802.
[http://dx.doi.org/10.1016/j.jnutbio.2012.04.013] [PMID: 22898567]

[71]   Sawatpanich T, Petpiboolthai H, Punyarachun B, Anupunpisit V. Effect of curcumin on vascular endothelial growth factor expression in diabetic mice kidney induced by streptozotocin. J Med Assoc Thai 2010; 93 (Suppl. 2): S1-8.
[PMID: 21302394]

[72]   Soetikno V, Watanabe K, Sari FR, *et al.* Curcumin attenuates diabetic nephropathy by inhibiting PKC-α and PKC-β1 activity in streptozotocin-induced type I diabetic rats. Mol Nutr Food Res 2011; 55(11): 1655-65.
[http://dx.doi.org/10.1002/mnfr.201100080] [PMID: 22045654]

[73]   Khajehdehi P, Pakfetrat M, Javidnia K, *et al.* Oral supplementation of turmeric attenuates proteinuria, transforming growth factor-β and interleukin-8 levels in patients with overt type 2 diabetic nephropathy: a randomized, double-blind and placebo-controlled study. Scand J Urol Nephrol 2011; 45(5): 365-70.
        [http://dx.doi.org/10.3109/00365599.2011.585622] [PMID: 21627399]

[74]   Farhangkhoee H, Khan ZA, Chen S, Chakrabarti S. Differential effects of curcumin on vasoactive factors in the diabetic rat heart. Nutr Metab (Lond) 2006; 3: 27.
        [http://dx.doi.org/10.1186/1743-7075-3-27] [PMID: 16848894]

[75]   Feng B, Chen S, Chiu J, George B, Chakrabarti S. Regulation of cardiomyocyte hypertrophy in diabetes at the transcriptional level. Am J Physiol Endocrinol Metab 2008; 294(6): E1119-26.
        [http://dx.doi.org/10.1152/ajpendo.00029.2008] [PMID: 18413674]

[76]   Hie M, Yamazaki M, Tsukamoto I. Curcumin suppresses increased bone resorption by inhibiting osteoclastogenesis in rats with streptozotocin-induced diabetes. Eur J Pharmacol 2009; 621(1-3): 1-9.
        [http://dx.doi.org/10.1016/j.ejphar.2009.08.025] [PMID: 19699734]

[77]   Cheng TC, Lin CS, Hsu CC, Chen LJ, Cheng KC, Cheng JT. Activation of muscarinic M-1 cholinoceptors by curcumin to increase glucose uptake into skeletal muscle isolated from Wistar rats. Neurosci Lett 2009; 465(3): 238-41.
        [http://dx.doi.org/10.1016/j.neulet.2009.09.012] [PMID: 19765405]

[78]   Na LX, Zhang YL, Li Y, *et al.* Curcumin improves insulin resistance in skeletal muscle of rats. Nutr Metab Cardiovasc Dis 2011; 21(7): 526-33.
        [http://dx.doi.org/10.1016/j.numecd.2009.11.009] [PMID: 20227862]

[79]   Deng YT, Chang TW, Lee MS, Lin JK. Suppression of free fatty acid-induced insulin resistance by phytopolyphenols in C2C12 mouse skeletal muscle cells. J Agric Food Chem 2012; 60(4): 1059-66.
        [http://dx.doi.org/10.1021/jf204496f] [PMID: 22191431]

[80]   Xavier S, Sadanandan J, George N, Paulose CS. β_2-adrenoceptor and insulin receptor expression in the skeletal muscle of streptozotocin induced diabetic rats: antagonism by vitamin D_3 and curcumin. Eur J Pharmacol 2012; 687(1-3): 14-20.
        [http://dx.doi.org/10.1016/j.ejphar.2012.02.050] [PMID: 22579915]

[81]   Abdel Aziz MT, Motawi T, Rezq A, *et al.* Effects of a water-soluble curcumin protein conjugate *vs.* pure curcumin in a diabetic model of erectile dysfunction. J Sex Med 2012; 9(7): 1815-33.
        [http://dx.doi.org/10.1111/j.1743-6109.2012.02741.x] [PMID: 22548787]

[82]   Kanter M, Aktas C, Erboga M. Curcumin attenuates testicular damage, apoptotic germ cell death, and oxidative stress in streptozotocin-induced diabetic rats. Mol Nutr Food Res 2013; 57(9): 1578-85.
        [http://dx.doi.org/10.1002/mnfr.201200170] [PMID: 22930655]

[83]   Jin QH, Shen HX, Wang H, Shou QY, Liu Q. Curcumin improves expression of SCF/c-kit through attenuating oxidative stress and NF-κB activation in gastric tissues of diabetic gastroparesis rats. Diabetol Metab Syndr 2013; 5(1): 12.
        [http://dx.doi.org/10.1186/1758-5996-5-12] [PMID: 23448582]

[84]   Qureshi M, Al-Suhaimi EA, Wahid F, Shehzad O, Shehzad A. Therapeutic potential of curcumin for multiple sclerosis. Neurol Sci 2018; 39(2): 207-14.
        [http://dx.doi.org/10.1007/s10072-017-3149-5] [PMID: 29079885]

[85]   Kamat AM, Sethi G, Aggarwal BB. Curcumin potentiates the apoptotic effects of chemotherapeutic agents and cytokines through down-regulation of nuclear factor-kappaB and nuclear factor-kappa--regulated gene products in IFN-alpha-sensitive and IFN-alpha-resistant human bladder cancer cells. Mol Cancer Ther 2007; 6(3): 1022-30.
        [http://dx.doi.org/10.1158/1535-7163.MCT-06-0545] [PMID: 17363495]

[86]   Shehzad A, Lee YS. Curcumin: Multiple molecular targets mediate multiple pharmacological actions. Drugs Future 2010; 35(2): 113-9.

[http://dx.doi.org/10.1358/dof.2010.035.02.1426640]

[87] Vrankova S, Parohova J, Barta A, Janega P, Simko F, Pechanova O. Effect of nuclear factor kappa B inhibition on L-NAME-induced hypertension and cardiovascular remodelling. J Hypertens 2010; 28 (Suppl. 1): S45-9.
[http://dx.doi.org/10.1097/01.hjh.0000388494.58707.0f] [PMID: 20823716]

[88] Nakmareong S, Kukongviriyapan U, Pakdeechote P, *et al.* Antioxidant and vascular protective effects of curcumin and tetrahydrocurcumin in rats with L-NAME-induced hypertension. Naunyn Schmiedebergs Arch Pharmacol 2011; 383(5): 519-29.
[http://dx.doi.org/10.1007/s00210-011-0624-z] [PMID: 21448566]

[89] Hlavačková L, Janegová A, Uličná O, Janega P, Cerná A, Babál P. Spice up the hypertension diet - curcumin and piperine prevent remodeling of aorta in experimental L-NAME induced hypertension. Nutr Metab (Lond) 2011; 8: 72.
[http://dx.doi.org/10.1186/1743-7075-8-72] [PMID: 22005253]

[90] Srinivasan K. Black pepper and its pungent principle-piperine: a review of diverse physiological effects. Crit Rev Food Sci Nutr 2007; 47(8): 735-48.
[http://dx.doi.org/10.1080/10408390601062054] [PMID: 17987447]

[91] Gardner DG. Natriuretic peptides: markers or modulators of cardiac hypertrophy? Trends Endocrinol Metab 2003; 14(9): 411-6.
[http://dx.doi.org/10.1016/S1043-2760(03)00113-9] [PMID: 14580760]

[92] Morimoto T, Sunagawa Y, Kawamura T, *et al.* The dietary compound curcumin inhibits p300 histone acetyltransferase activity and prevents heart failure in rats. J Clin Invest 2008; 118(3): 868-78.
[http://dx.doi.org/10.1172/JCI33160] [PMID: 18292809]

[93] Balasubramanyam K, Varier RA, Altaf M, *et al.* Curcumin, a novel p300/CREB-binding protein-specific inhibitor of acetyltransferase, represses the acetylation of histone/nonhistone proteins and histone acetyltransferase-dependent chromatin transcription. J Biol Chem 2004; 279(49): 51163-71.
[http://dx.doi.org/10.1074/jbc.M409024200] [PMID: 15383533]

[94] Sano M, Minamino T, Toko H, *et al.* p53-induced inhibition of Hif-1 causes cardiac dysfunction during pressure overload. Nature 2007; 446(7134): 444-8.
[http://dx.doi.org/10.1038/nature05602] [PMID: 17334357]

[95] Aggarwal BB, Shishodia S. Molecular targets of dietary agents for prevention and therapy of cancer. Biochem Pharmacol 2006; 71(10): 1397-421.
[http://dx.doi.org/10.1016/j.bcp.2006.02.009] [PMID: 16563357]

[96] Purcell NH, Tang G, Yu C, Mercurio F, DiDonato JA, Lin A. Activation of NF-kappa B is required for hypertrophic growth of primary rat neonatal ventricular cardiomyocytes. Proc Natl Acad Sci USA 2001; 98(12): 6668-73.
[http://dx.doi.org/10.1073/pnas.111155798] [PMID: 11381115]

[97] Manikandan P, Sumitra M, Aishwarya S, Manohar BM, Lokanadam B, Puvanakrishnan R. Curcumin modulates free radical quenching in myocardial ischaemia in rats. Int J Biochem Cell Biol 2004; 36(10): 1967-80.
[http://dx.doi.org/10.1016/j.biocel.2004.01.030] [PMID: 15203111]

[98] Bronte E, Coppola G, Di Miceli R, Sucato V, Russo A, Novo S. Role of curcumin in idiopathic pulmonary arterial hypertension treatment: a new therapeutic possibility. Med Hypotheses 2013; 81(5): 923-6.
[http://dx.doi.org/10.1016/j.mehy.2013.08.016] [PMID: 24054817]

[99] Rabinovitch M. Molecular pathogenesis of pulmonary arterial hypertension. J Clin Invest 2008; 118(7): 2372-9.
[http://dx.doi.org/10.1172/JCI33452] [PMID: 18596905]

[100] Schermuly RT, Ghofrani HA, Wilkins MR, Grimminger F. Mechanisms of disease: pulmonary arterial

hypertension. Nat Rev Cardiol 2011; 8(8): 443-55.
[http://dx.doi.org/10.1038/nrcardio.2011.87] [PMID: 21691314]

[101]   Zhou H, Beevers CS, Huang S. The targets of curcumin. Curr Drug Targets 2011; 12(3): 332-47.
[http://dx.doi.org/10.2174/138945011794815356] [PMID: 20955148]

[102]   Hajavi J, Momtazi AA, Johnston TP, Banach M, Majeed M, Sahebkar A. Curcumin: A naturally occurring modulator of adipokines in diabetes. J Cell Biochem 2017; 118(12): 4170-82.
[http://dx.doi.org/10.1002/jcb.26121] [PMID: 28485496]

[103]   Kelany ME, Hakami TM, Omar AH. Curcumin improves the metabolic syndrome in high-fructos--diet-fed rats: role of TNF-α, NF-κB, and oxidative stress. Can J Physiol Pharmacol 2017; 95(2): 140-50.
[http://dx.doi.org/10.1139/cjpp-2016-0152] [PMID: 27901349]

[104]   Jelodar G, Azimifar A. Evaluation of serum cancer antigen 125, resistin, leptin, homocysteine, and total antioxidant capacity in rat model of endometriosis treated with Curcumin. Physiol Rep 2019; 7(4)e14016
[http://dx.doi.org/10.14814/phy2.14016] [PMID: 30806992]

[105]   Rahimi HR, Mohammadpour AH, Dastani M, *et al.* The effect of nano-curcumin on HbA1c, fasting blood glucose, and lipid profile in diabetic subjects: a randomized clinical trial. Avicenna J Phytomed 2016; 6(5): 567-77.
[PMID: 27761427]

[106]   Abdel-Mageid AD, Abou-Salem MES, Salaam NMHA, El-Garhy HAS. The potential effect of garlic extract and curcumin nanoparticles against complication accompanied with experimentally induced diabetes in rats. Phytomedicine 2018; 43: 126-34.
[http://dx.doi.org/10.1016/j.phymed.2018.04.039] [PMID: 29747745]

[107]   Ganugula R, Arora M, Jaisamut P, *et al.* Nano-curcumin safely prevents streptozotocin-induced inflammation and apoptosis in pancreatic beta cells for effective management of Type 1 diabetes mellitus. Br J Pharmacol 2017; 174(13): 2074-84.
[http://dx.doi.org/10.1111/bph.13816] [PMID: 28409821]

[108]   Nishizono S, Hayami T, Ikeda I, Imaizumi K. Protection against the diabetogenic effect of feeding tert-butylhydroquinone to rats prior to the administration of streptozotocin. Biosci Biotechnol Biochem 2000; 64(6): 1153-8.
[http://dx.doi.org/10.1271/bbb.64.1153] [PMID: 10923784]

CHAPTER 3

Olive Leaf: A Traditional Phytomedicine for Diabetes and Hypertension

José Luis Ríos[1,*], Isabel Andújar[1,2], Luisa González-Arbeláez[3], Guillermo R. Schinella[4,5] and Flavio Francini[6]

[1] *Departament de Farmacologia, Facultat de Farmacia, Universitat de València, Burjassot, Spain*

[2] *Departamento de Ciencias Biomédicas. Universidad Europea de Valencia, Valencia, Spain*

[3] *Centro de Investigaciones Cardiovasculares, CCT UNLP-CONICET, La Plata, Argentina*

[4] *Cátedra de Farmacología Básica. Facultad de Ciencias Médicas, UNLP, La Plata, Argentina*

[5] *Instituto de Ciencias de la Salud - CICPBA, Universidad Nacional Arturo Jauretche, Florencio Varela, Argentina*

[6] *CENEXA; UNLP-CONICET CCT La Plata-FCM; CEAS-CICPBA, La Plata, Argentina*

Abstract: Olive leaves are used in Mediterranean folk medicine for the treatment of diabetes, hypertension, and hypercholesterolemia since ancient times. In the last decade, different authors have studied their chemical composition and ratified their pharmacological properties both *in vitro* and *in vivo*, and, more recently, clinical trials focusing on their effects on diabetes and hypertension have been developed. Oleuropein and hydroxytyrosol seem to emerge as promising bioactive phenolics responsible for these beneficial effects. In this chapter, information about recent studies on the olive leaf is compiled, including its effects on the specific subject of this chapter, but also its other potential pharmacological effects.

Keywords: Antidiabetic, Antihypertensive, Hydroxytyrosol, Hypoglycemic, *Olea europaea*, Oleuropeoside.

INTRODUCTION

According to the last revision of The Plant List [1], the Oleaceae family includes 25 accepted and 7 unassessed genera. The genus *Olea* comprises 35 accepted species and, among them, *Olea europaea* L. has the highest relevance. Classically, about 10 varieties and 4 subspecies were described, but, at present, all of them are considered synonyms of *Olea europaea* L., the only taxon accepted [1]. This species is widely known and used for its fruits and the oil obtained from

---

[*] **Corresponding autor José Luis Ríos:** Departament de Farmacologia, Facultat de Farmacia, Universitat de València, Av. Vicent Andrés Estellés s/n, 46100 Burjassot, Spain; Tel: +34 963544973; E-mail: rios@uv.es

them in the Mediterranean diet [2]. *Olea europaea* is included in the taxonomical group of flowering plants (Spermatophyta) and the class of dicotyledons (Magnoliopsida). The whole taxonomy is compiled in Table **1** according to the United States Department of Agriculture classification [3].

Table 1. Taxonomy of *Olea europaea* [3].

Biological Group	Taxonomy	Common Name
Kingdom	Plantae	Plants
Subkingdom	Tracheobionta	Vascular plants
Superdivision	Spermatophyta	Seed plants
Division	Magnoliophyta	Flowering plants
Class	Magnoliopsida	Dicotyledons
Subclass	Asteridae	
Order	Scrophulariales	
Family	Oleaceae	Olive family
Genus	*Olea* L.	Olive
Species	*Olea europaea* L.	Olive

The olive tree is an evergreen tree (Fig. **1**) or shrub of variable height (8-15 m) and diameter, depending on the kind of olive, variety, age of the tree, and if it grows wild or cultivated. The leaves have about 4-10 cm length, 1-3 cm width, and are pale green with few scales on the top, and silvery-whitish at the below. The fruit is an ovoid drupe, blackish-violet when ripe, normally of 1.0-2.5 cm long, smaller in wild plants than in orchard cultivates. It has a central pit that encloses the seed surrounded by the edible fleshy mesocarp. Genetically, an olive tree is a diploid species [4, 5].

Olive trees are distributed along the Mediterranean coast, including southeastern Europe, northern Iran (south end of the Caspian Sea), western Asia, and North Africa. The fruit and leaves of the olive tree are also important in the context of religion because they are cited in both New and Old Testaments [4]. The principal producer of olives and olive oil is Spain, followed by Italy and Greece, whereas, out of Europe, the United States of America and Argentina are the major producers [4 - 6]. The cultivation of olive dates goes back to more than 7000 years for commercial purposes in Crete, Greece, and the Middle East, and from where it was spread to the West to the Italian and Iberian peninsulas, as well as France. It reached the American continent with Spaniards when they arrived in Peru, Mexico, and California [4]. The olive tree is a typical component of the thermo-Mediterranean climate; it is a thermophile species adapted to tolerate drought and salinity stress and grows on a wide range of soils [5].

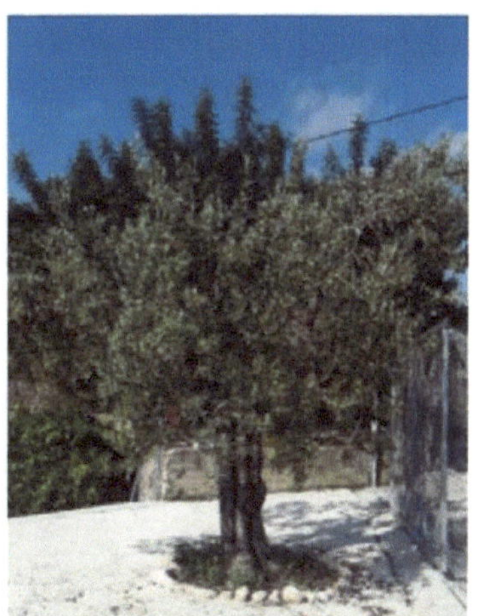 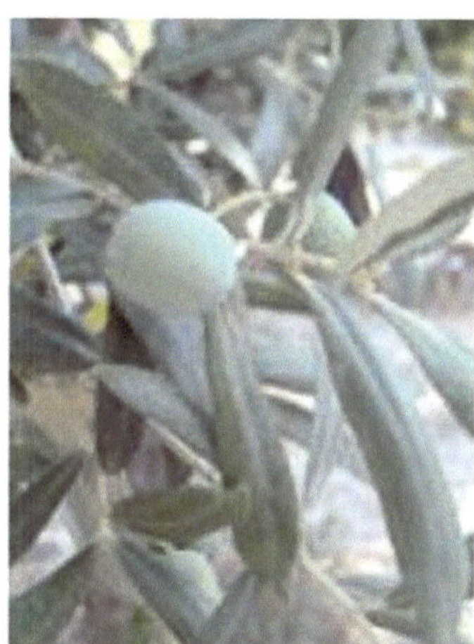

Fig. (1). *Olea europaea*. The olive tree, leaves, and fruits.

OLIVE, A MEDITERRANEAN TREE WITH A HIGH VALUE FOR ECONOMY AND HEALTH

The olive tree is probably the most economically important crop tree of the Mediterranean region [5]. It is appreciated for its wood [7], fruits [8], and oil [9]. The olive tree wood is heavy and very tough, and it is usually employed for manufacturing high-end furniture, inlays, turned objects, and handcrafts [5, 7]. It is also appreciated as firewood because it burns even when wet and to obtain charcoal [5, 7, 10]. The fruit is edible after processing because the natural fruits are extremely bitter and need a process for reducing the bitterness. This process usually includes soaking the fruits in salt-water to make them more palatable, processing them with NaOH, or drying them in the sun [8]. Pickled, canned, or otherwise prepared table olives are eaten as a relish or used in bread, salads, or other preparations [5]. In the case of olive oil, its principal use is as food (in crude) or for cooking, but other relevant uses make this oil of high interest [11]. Its uses include medical and pharmaceutical use as well as for ointments, lighting (burning without smoke), and medical uses [5, 9]. Virgin olive oil is the principal component of the Mediterranean diet, and it is of a high value for its beneficial properties for human health due to the high amounts of unsaturated fatty acids [5]. Mediterranean countries produce more than 77% of the olive oil in the world, with Spain (36%), Italy (24%) and Greece (17%) being the major producers, whereas 17.4% oil is from the Mediterranean countries of Africa, and the rest of the world produces 5.6% of the total production [9].

Finally, other products of olive can be of interest, mainly the leaves, which are used in medicine as a herbal tea for their high content in phenolics, especially oleuropein and hydroxytyrosol. Olive is also used in gardens as an ornamental tree and as a bonsai tree [5].

CHEMICAL COMPOSITION OF OLIVE LEAF

Olive leaves contain different groups of phytochemicals: secoiridoids, flavonoids and other phenolics, steroids and triterpenes, and other compounds, whereas triglycerides and other lipophilic compounds are present in oil from seeds. Hashmi *et al.* [4], reviewed the chemical composition of olive and described 140 compounds, with secoiridoids, being the principal group with about 40 compounds followed by the different groups of phenolics (ethyl and propyl derivatives, flavonoids, and lignans). Among them, about 30 compounds were isolated from different leave extracts. Another relevant review is the one published by Talhaoui *et al.* [6], in the same year, which included other complementary compounds also isolated from the leaves, among which oleuropein (Fig. **2**) stands out. Other relevant secoiridoids and related compounds cited by these authors include oleuropein aglycone, oleuropein glucoside, demethyloleuropein, methoxyoleuropein, lingstroside, oleuricine A, elenolic acid methyl ester, hydroxytyrosil-elenolate, oleoside, secologanoside, comselogoside, oleuricine B, oleuroside, 6β-*O*-[(2*E*)-2,6-dimethyl-8-hydroxy-2-octeno-loxy]-secologanoside, and oleacein as the main secoiridoids; compound 4'-*O*-β-D-glucosyl-9-O-(6"-deoxysaccharosyl)olivil as representative oflignans; the flavonoidsapigenin, apigenin-7-*O*-glucoside, apigenin-7-*O*-rutinoside, luteolin, luteolin-7-*O*-glucoside, luteolin-7, 4'-*O*-diglucoside, quercetin, rutin, quercetrin, diosmetin, chrysoeriol-7-*O*-glucoside, and catechin; the phenolics, tyrosol, tyrosol glucoside, hydroxytyrosol, hydroxytyrosol glucoside, verbascoside, isoverbascosideand vanillin; the organic acids vanillic, caffeic, gallic, cinnamic, hydroxycinammic, syringic, ferulic, *p*-hydroxybenzoic, chlorogenic, protocatechic, and hydroxyphenylacetic; the triterpenoids erythrodiol, uvaol, ursolic acid, maslinic acid, β-amyrin, urs-2β, 3β-dihydroxy-12-en-28-oic acid, and betulinic acid; the sterol sitosterol; and the only monosaccharide derivative isolated from this species, 1,5-anhydroxylitol [4, 6].

Some lipophilic compounds have been described to be present in the leaves, such as myristic, palmitic, stearic, oleic, linoleic, linolenic, and arachidic acids [12]. The same authors also described the presence of different trace elements in concentrations that range from 11448 µg/g for K to 0.14 µg/g for Cr. They described the contents of proteins, lipids, and carbohydrates, which vary depending on the variety of olive, but on average, we can consider 7.7% of proteins, 2.6% of lipids, and 36.3% of carbohydrates [7, 12].

Oleuropein

Hydroxytyrosol

Rutin

Oleanolic acid

Fig. (2). Examples of relevant molecules present in olive leaves.

PHARMACOLOGICAL PROPERTIES

To summarize, olive leaves are a sub-product of olive tree cultivation and relevant amounts of leaves are collected during pruning, harvest, and processing, therefore they can be considered a cheap source of high added-value phenolic compounds with a potential role in phytomedicine, cosmetics, and functional foods [13].

In folk medicine, olive leaves are usually employed alone or in combination with other medicinal plants. For example, decoctions of dried leaves are used to treat diarrhea, respiratory and urinary tract infections, stomach and intestinal diseases, and as mouth cleanser [4]. However, the main use of the leaves' extract is the treatment of high blood pressure [14 - 20] and diabetes [7, 17 - 20]. Other uses of interest are in inflammatory disorders, infections, and digestive tract disorders. To increase the knowledge of these potential pharmacological actions, different studies have been carried out, which have demonstrated their antioxidant, hypocholesterolemic, and anti-inflammatory activities [21]. Among the different actions described for the leaves' extracts, their antioxidant properties are also linked to its anti-inflammatory effects, especially in inflammatory disorders such as ulcerative colitis. Ferreira *et al.* [22], Benavente-García *et al.* [23], Silva *et al.* [24], and others investigated the potentiality of phenolics from olive leaves as antioxidants and established the interest for both the extract and the isolated compounds, which have a synergistic effect with higher antioxidant capacity than the biological references, vitamins C and E [21].

One relevant property of olive leaf is its hypocholesterolemic effect because it reduces triglycerides by 23% (1 g extract/d) and low-density lipoprotein (LDL)-cholesterol levels [25]. Studies carried out in animals demonstrated that the leaf extract reduces blood levels of total cholesterol, triglycerides, and LDL-cholesterol, and increased high-density lipoprotein (HDL)-cholesterol [26]. Other studies were performed with isolated active principles and, in this case, administration of oleuropein (10-20 mg/kg) for 6 weeks reduced both total cholesterol and triglycerides in hypercholesterolemic rabbits [27]. The administration of an enriched-extract with oleuropein (8 and 16 mg/kg) or hydroxytyrosol (8 and 16 mg/kg) also reduced total cholesterol in about 37% in diabetic rats, restoring normal values (non-treated rats) [28]. In conclusion, olive leaf phenolics can reduce the levels of triglycerides and cholesterol–total and LDL– increasing HDL-cholesterol.

Another relevant property of olive leaf phenolics is their anti-inflammatory activity, which was demonstrated in different experimental models. For example, oleuropein (20 mg/kg, ip, immediately and 1 h after spinal cord injury) reduces levels of tumor necrosis factor (TNF)-α, interleukin (IL)-1β, and nitrotyrosine, as well as the expression of inducible nitric oxide synthase (iNOS), cyclooxygenase-2 (COX-2), and poly (ADP-ribose) polymerase (PARP) in treated-rats, respect to the trauma control [29]. Oral administration of oleuropein (40 mg/mouse/d for 8 days) attenuated the acute colitis symptoms (extent and severity) induced by dextran sulfate sodium, with reduction of neutrophil infiltration, NO, IL-1β, IL-6, and TNF-α production, expression of iNOS, COX-2, and matrix metalloproteinase 9 (MMP-9), and nuclear translocation of nuclear factor (NF)-κB p65 subunit [30]. These same authors assayed oleuropein (500 mg/kg, p.o., 56 days) on an experimental model of chronic colitis induced by dextran sulfate sodium and observed that it decreased the release of pro-inflammatory cytokines (IL-1β and IL-6) and reduced inflammatory cells migration to the inflamed tissue [31]. In summary, the anti-inflammatory effect of oleuropein is associated with a decrease in the production of pro-inflammatory mediators, such as interleukins and reduced expression of pro-inflammatory enzymes, mainly through the reduction of NF-κB activation.

The references to the anticancer or antitumoral properties are not to be considered, because the publications are focused on the cytotoxic properties on different cancer cell lines [4], but no relevant studies are carried out on animals (antitumoral) or humans (anticancer). In the case of the antimicrobial activity, some interesting results have been published, but no the minimum inhibitory concentration of extracts or principles is reported. Different papers published the inhibition halos against fungi [32] or bacteria [33], with some interest for the aqueous extract.

ANTIHYPERTENSIVE PROPERTIES OF OLIVE LEAF

The increase of hypertension worldwide is a major global health challenge because it is the main cause of cardiovascular and kidney diseases and the principal responsibility of the increase of morbidity and mortality in humans, as well as the first reason for the increase of financial costs for the health system. The values of the prevalence of hypertension around the world are very different, but they increased in the last decades. As an example, the lowest prevalence in rural India is about 3.4% in men and 6.8% in women, whereas the highest prevalence is for people of Poland, with values of 68.9% in men and 72.5% in women [34, 35]. In 2018, the task force formed by the European Society of Cardiology and the European Society of Hypertension defined hypertension as a systolic blood pressure of 140 mmHg or more, or diastolic blood pressure of 90 mmHg or more [36]. On the other hand, in the following guidelines issued by the American Heart Association, hypertension is defined as blood pressure higher than 130 over 80 mmHg [37].

The strategies for hypertension treatment include in a first step changes in lifestyle, such as salt restriction, moderation of alcohol consumption, high consumption of vegetables and fruits, weight reduction, maintaining ideal body weight, regular physical activity, and smoking cessation [36]. However, many patients will require pharmacological treatment in addition to lifestyle measures to achieve optimal blood pressure control. Five major drug classes were recommended for the treatment of hypertension: angiotensin-converting enzyme inhibitors, angiotensin receptor blockers, beta-blockers, calcium channel blockers, and thiazide diuretics are suitable for the initiation and maintenance of antihypertensive treatment, alone or in combination [36, 37].

In cases where treatment of hypertension is required with complementary therapies, such as phytotherapy, there are different species with potential interest [38, 39], among which the olive leaf stands out. This interest is reinforced by the fact that the traditional Mediterranean diet is epidemiologically associated with long life and a lower prevalence of cardiovascular diseases and cancers because the diet is rich in olive derivatives [40]. This knowledge is supported by several preclinical studies using different experimental models, which have shown the potential health benefits of olive oil and olive leaf extract and natural products isolated from them. There are many studies *in vitro* and *in vivo* on the antihypertensive effects of olive leaf extracts [41], which could validate the interest for their studies in humans [42]. For that, this review aimed to present the main publications of clinical studies with extracts or natural products isolated from olive leaves in the treatment of hypertension.

Among other epidemiological studies, in the large European Prospective Investigation into Cancer and Nutrition study with 20343 subjects had never received a diagnosis of hypertension, and the Prevention with Mediterranean Diet trial with 7447 patients with a high risk for cardiovascular disease, the intake of extra-virgin olive oil, rich in polyphenols, was inversely associated with both systolic blood pressure and diastolic blood pressure [43, 44]. Not only the olive oil was used, but the leaves have also been used for medical purposes. In several clinical studies, olive leaf extract induced reductions of blood pressure. For example, a preliminary clinical study carried out in patients suffering from essential hypertension (12 patients consulting for the first time, and 18 patients with antihypertensive treatment) received 400 mg extract ×4/day for 3 months. All of them had a statistically significant decrease in blood pressure [45]. Recently, different clinical trials were carried out and differ in their study protocols; they are summarized in Table **2**.

A recent study evaluated the effects of olive leaf extract on metabolic response and biomarkers of inflammation in a randomized, double-blind placebo-controlled clinical trial with hypertensive patients (30-60 years, n=60) who received either extract (250 mg) or placebo tablets for 12 weeks. Changes in parameters associated with glucose metabolism were not statistically significant in the extract group; however, the extract decreased IL-6, IL-8, and TNF-α compared to the placebo group. These results concluded that olive leaf extract decreased the pro-inflammatory mediators, but had no effects associated with glucose metabolism [50].

The mechanisms underlying these antihypertensive effects were observed in preclinical models, and they may involve the inhibition of angiotensin-converting enzyme and/or calcium channel blockers activities [51 - 54]. When the influence of polyphenol from olive on hypertensive patients was investigated in clinical trials, the reduction of pressure was attributed to the improvement of endothelial function [55, 56] and the modulation of the expression of some of the genes related to the renin-angiotensin-aldosterone system [48, 57]. Also, the olive leaf extract and polyphenol-rich olive oil improved the plasmatic cholesterol in patients with pre-hypertensive and stage-1 hypertension [45, 49]. Both the antihypertensive and cholesterol-lowering properties could be beneficial for reducing the risk of cardiovascular diseases. Besides, the olive leaf extract should also be investigated for its effects on pro-inflammatory mediators, which are the major cause of hypertension.

Table 2. Relevant clinical trials carried out with olive leaf extract.

Authors (Year)	Study Type and Conditions	N, sex (F/M) Age Duration	Kind of Extract and Dose	Observed Effect	Ref
Perrinjaquet-Moccetti *et al.* (2008)	OL, PG Pre-hypertensive monozygotic twins	40 (28/12) 18-20 8 wk	Standardized extract 250 mg ×2/d or 500 mg ×2/d, equivalent to 52 or 104 mg oleuropein/d	At 1000 mg/d an anti-hypertensive effect was confirmed	[46]
Susalit *et al.* (2011)	DB, CR Stage-1 hypertension	148 (126/22) 25-60 8 wk	Standardized extract 500 mg ×2/d, equivalent to 104 mg oleuropein/d	At 1000 mg/d lowered systolic and diastolic blood pressures similar to captopril	[25]
de Bock *et al.* (2013)	DB, CR Overweight and normotension	45 (0/45) 35-55 12 wk	Extract equivalent (51.1 mg Oleuropein + 9.7 mg hydroxytyrosol)/d	Supplementation with extract did not modify 24-h ambulatory blood pressure	[47]
Cabrera-Vique *et al.* (2015)	NR Pre-hypertension	10 (NR/NR) NR 28 d	Extract (400 mg ×4/d), equivalent (240 mg oleuropein + 1.6 mg hydroxytyrosol)/d	There was a decrease in the diastolic and systolic pressure	[48]
Lockyer *et al.* (2017)	DB, CR Pre-hypertension	60 (0/60 18-65 6 wk	Extract equivalent (136 mg oleuropein + 6 mg hydroxytyrosol)/d	Extract intake engenders hypotension	[49]

CR, crossover; d, day; DB, double-blind; F, female; M, male; N, number of patients; NR, not reported; OL, open-label; PG, parallel-group; wk, week.

ANTIHYPERGLYCEMIC PROPERTIES OF OLIVE LEAF

Type 2 Diabetes Mellitus (T2D) is a chronic disease that, if not treated and controlled properly, generates severe disabling complications and, therefore, raises the economic cost becoming a serious burden for Public Health [58]. Worldwide, care of T2D patients consumes between 5 to 10% of the budget allocated to the health system due to a higher frequency of consultations and hospitalizations, and longer re-hospitalizations and complexity of the treatments [59]. Its prevalence is constantly increasing worldwide, and different studies predict that in the next years, there will be a dramatic increase in the number of patients worldwide [60]. T2D is characterized by a state of hyperglycemia, because of metabolic disorders resulting from a defect in insulin secretion by pancreatic β-cells, an increase in peripheral resistance to this hormone, or both

[61]. The evidence indicates that there is no diabetes without the existence of β-cell failure. Faced with inadequate or poor glycemic control, the patient can start a chronic process leading to a multiorgan failure affecting the eye, kidney, vessels, and heart, and inducing associated negative processes to other risks, such as hypertension, dyslipidemia or overweight [61]. The increase of glucose levels, consecutive to food intake, leads to an increase in the uptake of sugar by pancreatic β-cells and their subsequent metabolism within it. Once glucose is metabolized, it increases the ATP/ADP ratio in the β-cell and this leads to remodeling ion fluxes at the plasma membrane, which culminates in stimulating insulin secretion. Released insulin reaches through the bloodstream its receptor in different peripheral tissues activating the signal responsible for its metabolic effects: carbohydrate uptake and storage, or lipid synthesis which results in increasing lipogenesis. As mentioned in the first paragraphs, alterations in circulating levels of insulin are due to two processes: an alteration in their secretion because of the alteration of the hormone-producing cells and a decrease or loss of response of the peripheral tissues, a phenomenon known as insulin resistance [62]. In an insulin-resistant cell, the signal transduction that triggers the hormone deteriorates and, therefore, the endocrine-metabolic effects that it should exert on that cell. Likewise, an inflammatory process begins.

The impaired β-cell function can be associated with three different causes: a decrease in sensitivity to glucose, loss of pulses, and the biphasic pattern of insulin secretion, and a decrease in β-cell mass. In the first case, the sensitivity of β-cells to glucose decreases progressively from a state of impaired glucose tolerance to T2D [63]. On the other hand, biphasic profile and pulses are altered at the early stages of T2D, thus becoming good markets of the progressive decline in the cell function. Finally, an adequate β-cell mass is essential for controlling glycemic control and preventing the development of T2D. In this sense, clinical studies evinced in T2D patients had an imbalance between the rate of cell renewal and apoptosis, showing a 50-60% decrease in β-cell mass [64]. This fact is also evident in the early stages of the development of T2D, like impaired glucose tolerance [65]. Interestingly, hyperglycemia plays a key role in impairing insulin secretion and β-cell mass (glucotoxicity) associated with a process of oxidative stress-related DNA damage in the islet of patients with T2D [66]. The higher demand for insulin secretion under an insulin-resistant scenario leads to a functional overload of β-cells that could be responsible for the activation of endoplasmic reticulum stress and that leads to apoptosis *via* C/EBP homologous protein induction [67]. These results highlight the importance of chronic ER stress in beta-cell apoptosis in type 2 diabetes and suggest a new target to the management of the disease.

The development of T2D in patients with impaired glucose tolerance can be prevented or delayed by the implementation of lifestyle changes and healthy nutrition, weight reduction, and physical activity [68] or by several drugs administration [69 - 71]. However, those patients where the functionality in the β-cells has been lost, treatment with insulin is required. Complementary and alternatives therapies such as herbal medicine have been used since ancient times. In our days, even when these therapies are long-standing in Easter cultures, they are employed all around the world, especially in those patients where conventional medicine fails to improve diseases. Consequently, it is worth asking if herbal medicine can help to control and improve the quality of life of the patient with T2D or eventually, delay or avoid pharmacological treatment. In this context, different drugs have been used to treat T2D, and some of them are incorporated as therapeutic tools to treat the illness. Several of these compounds are natural products that have been obtained from plants or microbes and were recently revised by Ríos *et al.* [72]. Among them, extracts, herbal teas, and powder from olive leaves have been used [41, 42]. These preparations contain bioactive compounds that can act as antioxidants, anti-inflammatory, antihypertensive, antiatherogenic, and hypoglycaemic agents. Even when several compounds could account for the protective effect of olive derivatives, recent research has focused on their polyphenols, as mentioned previously, to which the mentioned beneficial actions have been ascribed [73].

While in an *in vitro* study, leaf and olive fruit extract rich in oleuropein protects INS-1 cells from the deleterious effect of cytokines [74], several studies in animal models have evinced the antidiabetic and hypolipidemic effects of olive leaves [75]. Al-Azzawie and Alhamdani treated hypoglycemic alloxan-diabetic rabbits with oleuropein (20 mg/Kg body weight) for up to 16 weeks and they observed that, together with an improvement of antioxidant content, blood glucose levels were comparable to normal control rabbits [76]. These studies have identified some phenolic compounds of alcoholic extract such as oleuropein and hydroxytyrosol as responsible for the hypocholesterolaemia and hypoglycaemic effects. Jemai *et al.* [28], provoked in rats hyperglycemia, increased lipid peroxidation and oxidative stress together with hypercholesterolemia, and they demonstrated that administration of oleuropein and hydroxytyrosol rich extracts (8–16 mg/kg body weight of each compound) for 4 weeks restored basal serum cholesterol and glucose levels. In another study, streptozotocin-diabetic rats were orally administered with olive leaves extracts (100, 250, and 500 mg/kg of body weight) and glibenclamide (600 μg/kg) as a reference drug, for 14 days, demonstrating a more potent effect with the olive leaves extract than glibenclamide. On the other hand, 100 mg/kg/day of oleanolic acid when administered during 7 days to diabetic high fat-fed mice, clearly decreased plasma glucose and insulin levels, and improved glucose tolerance after an intraperitoneal glucose tolerance test [77].

Additionally, together with the lowering of serum glucose activities, the extract increased insulinemia in diabetic but not in normal rats [78]. More recently, Dubey *et al.* [79] demonstrated the protective effect of oleanolic acid on streptozotocin-induced diabetic neuropathy in Sprague Dawley rats, when these rats were treated daily with different doses of oleanolic acid (20, 40, and 60 mg/Kg) up to four weeks.

Oleuropein effects have been ascribed to different molecular mechanisms: improvement in glucose-induced insulin release and increase in peripheral glucose uptake reducing then plasma glucose levels [80]. Additionally, Bennani-Kabchi *et al.* [81], demonstrated in obese prediabetic rats (*Psammomys obesus*) a hypocholesterolemia effect (42%) related to a decrease in LDL and VLDL. These effects were not accompanied by a parallel decrease in plasma levels of triglycerides and HDL-cholesterol. More recently, evaluating the effects of an ethanolic extract of olive leaves on the metabolism of diabetic rats (induced by a high-fat diet and low dose of streptozotocin), it was demonstrated that ethanolic extract of olive leaves at doses of 200 and 400 mg/kg during 10 weeks induced a significant decrease in body weight and an improvement in glucose levels in diabetic animals compared to diabetic untreated rats [82].

However, in humans, even when several trials have been performed with natural products therapies, few of them address a possible beneficial effect of olive tree leaves derivatives on metabolic alterations and especially on glucose homeostasis [83] even when olive leaf infusion is widely used as a folk medicine to treat diabetes [80].

In a study, five 32-68 years old male patient diagnosed with T1D under recurrent insulin treatment were administrated with a hydroxytyrosol-concentrated extract obtained from olive oil wastewaters, composed of hydroxytyrosol (53%) and tyrosol (13%) in the free form and elenolic acid and derivatives (34%). Hydroxytyrosol content was adjusted to 10 mg/ml. The preparation was administrated together with yogurt containing either 25 mg (first day, T_0, baseline) or 12.5 mg hydroxytyrosol (at time points 1, 2, 3, and 4 h after T_0.) for 4 days [84]. After that period glycemia and HbA1c, indicatives of diabetic status were not modified by the treatment. However, a significant decrease in thromboxane B_2 release was found. Even when glycemia was not modified, this result could be of interest in the context of thrombosis prevention in diabetic patients, as the authors stated [84].

In a randomized, double-blind, placebo-controlled clinical trial, 79 patients diagnosed with T2D (18-79 years old; 51/28 male/female) were randomized into two groups: patients treated with a tablet of olive leaf extract (500 mg) or placebo taken orally once daily for 14 weeks. In those patients treated with olive leaf extract, HbA1c levels were reduced significantly when compared to placebo. This effect was accompanied by a significant decrease in fasting insulinemia without changes in glycemia [80].

Finally, in a crossover trial, 46 overweight men (BMI 25-30 kg/m^2), aged 35-55 years old, were randomized using computer random number generation, to receive olive leaf extract capsules or placebo for 12 weeks [47]. The patients administered a daily dose of 51.1 mg oleuropein and 9.7 mg hydroxytyrosol. Then the volunteers were switched over to the other treatment after a 6 weeks washout period and once again a 12 weeks intervention. Olive leaf extract supplementation induced a 15% improvement in insulin sensitivity and this change was related to a 28% improvement in pancreatic β-cell function. Additionally, the beneficial effect was also observed in a reduction of the area under the curve for both glucose and insulin, without changes in the lipid profile.

The association of olive leaf polyphenols with fenugreek and bergamot extract did not improve the glucose homeostasis in patients with prediabetes. The assay was performed as a single-center, randomized, double-blind, placebo-controlled trial; patients with prediabetes (n=100, for 6 months) [85].

A drawback in the determination of the clinical relevance of many of the animals and *in vitro* experiments is the uncertainty about the correlation of those results with the end effects in humans. An example that highlights this is the study carried out by Pyner *et al.* [86]. These authors analyzed the acute effects of olive leaf extract and an oleuropein-enriched extract on sucrase activity both *in vitro* and *in vivo*. Long-term pre-treatment *in vitro* with the enriched-fraction of olive leaf extract lowered sucrose-isomaltase activity and attenuated subsequent sucrose hydrolysis. However, in a randomized, double-blinded, placebo-controlled, crossover pilot study with 50 mg oleuropein 3 times a day for 1 week (healthy young women, n=11), changes in post-prandial blood glucose were not appreciated, concluding that changes in sucrose-isomaltase activity are not sufficient to induce functional effects in healthy volunteers [86]. Although current studies carried out *in vitro* or animals are promising, they have many inconsistencies; for example, the extracts were obtained through different systems such as maceration, Soxhlet, and supercritical fluid extraction methods. Besides, different solvents (ethanol, methanol) were used, and the standardized extracts were evaluated in different components (oleuropein, hydroxytyrosol, luteolin). Finally, the doses were also variable [87]. Therefore, they should only be considered as complementary.

DISCUSSION AND FUTURE PERSPECTIVES

In general, the establishment of the efficacy of plant products is limited by the number of clinical trials, the reduced number of patients, and the diversification in the standardization of the samples. In the case of the antihypertensive effect of olive, many studies have been carried out *in vitro* and *in vivo* with olive leaf extracts and with polyphenols from extra-virgin olive oil (also present in the leaves). Clinical studies performed with olive leaf extract demonstrate a reduction in blood pressure. The mechanism implicated in this effect was established using preclinical models concluding that the inhibition of angiotensin-converting enzyme and/or calcium channel blockers activities are implicated. Clinical studies with hypertensive patients showed that the reduction of pressure was related to the improvement of endothelial function and the modulation of the expression of some of the genes related to the renin-angiotensin-aldosterone system. Besides, the olive leaf extract and polyphenol-rich olive oil-modified the plasmatic cholesterolemia in pre-hypertensive patients and patients with stage-1 hypertension. Both the antihypertensive and cholesterol-lowering properties are implicated in the protection against cardiovascular disease and would justify the use of olive with this aim in folk medicine.

In the case of T2D, the olive oil extracts have bioactive phenolics, antioxidant, anti-inflammatory, antihypertensive and antiatherogenic, and hypoglycaemic activities. Even when several compounds could account for the protective effect of olive derivatives, recent research has focused on oleuropein and hydroxytyrosol, to which the mentioned beneficial actions have been ascribed. Several *in vivo* studies with oleuropein-rich leaf and olive fruit extracts evidenced antidiabetic and hypolipidemic properties, identifying oleuropein and hydroxytyrosol as responsible for the hypocholesterolaemic and hypoglycaemic effects. However, in the performed clinical trials, limited effects on metabolic alterations, and especially on glucose homeostasis have been reported. Clinical trials in patients treated with olive leaf extract demonstrated a significant reduction of HbA1c levels *vs.* placebo, with a decrease in fasting insulinemia, but with no changes in glycemia. Nevertheless, when extracts or enriched foods were used in the clinical trials, no modifications in glycemia or HbA1c were detected. Interestingly, a clear decrease in thromboxane B_2 release was observed, which can be of interest for the prevention of thrombosis in diabetic patients. Finally, the treatment of overweight men with olive leaf extract proved to induce a 15% improvement in insulin sensitivity, and this change was associated with the improvement in pancreatic β-cell function, and a reduction of the area under the curve for both glucose and insulin.

In conclusion, more randomized controlled human clinical trials with standardized extracts, and extensive toxicity studies are needed to evaluate potential health effects and safety of olive leaves.

CONSENT FOR PUBLICATION

Not applicable.

CONFLICT OF INTEREST

There is no conflict of interest declared.

ACKNOWLEDGEMENT

Declared none.

REFERENCES

[1]   http://www.theplantlist.org/1.1/browse/A/Oleaceae/Olea/

[2]   Julca I, Marcet-Houben M, Vargas P, Gabaldón T. Phylogenomics of the olive tree (*Olea europaea*) reveals the relative contribution of ancient allo- and autopolyploidization events. BMC Biol 2018; 16(1): 15.
[http://dx.doi.org/10.1186/s12915-018-0482-y] [PMID: 29370802]

[3]   Natural Resources Conservation Service https://plants.usda.gov/java/ClassificationServlet?source= profile&symbol=OLEU&display=31

[4]   Hashmi MA, Khan A, Hanif M, Farooq U, Perveen S. Traditional uses phytochemistry and pharmacology of *Olea europaea* (olive). Evid Based Complement Alternat Med 2015; 2015541591
[http://dx.doi.org/10.1155/2015/541591] [PMID: 25802541]

[5]   Guerrero-Maldonado N, López MJ, Caudullu G, de Rigo D. Olea europaea in Europe: distribution, habitat, usage and threats.European Atlas of Forest Tree Species. Luxembourg: Publ Off EU 2016; p. e01534b.

[6]   Talhaoui N, Taamalli A, Gómez-Caravaca AM, Fernández-Gutiérrez A, Segura-Carretero A. Phenolic compounds in olive leaves: Analytical determination, biotic and abiotic influence, and health benefits. Food Res Int 2015; 77: 92-108.
[http://dx.doi.org/10.1016/j.foodres.2015.09.011]

[7]   Terral JF. Exploitation and management of the olive tree during prehistoric times in Mediterranean France and Spain. J Archaeol Sci 2000; 27: 127-33.
[http://dx.doi.org/10.1006/jasc.1999.0444]

[8]   Kailis S, Harris D. Producing table olives. Collingwood, Australia: Landlinks Press 2007.
[http://dx.doi.org/10.1071/9780643094383]

[9]   Vossen P. Olive oil: history, production, and characteristics world's classic oils. HortScience 2007; 42: 1093-100.
[http://dx.doi.org/10.21273/HORTSCI.42.5.1093]

[10]   Breton C, Terral JF, Pinatel C, Médail F, Bonhomme F, Bervillé A. The origins of the domestication of the olive tree. C R Biol 2009; 332(12): 1059-64.
[http://dx.doi.org/10.1016/j.crvi.2009.08.001] [PMID: 19931842]

[11]   Besnard G, Terral JF, Cornille A. On the origins and domestication of the olive: a review and perspectives. Ann Bot 2018; 121(3): 385-403.
[http://dx.doi.org/10.1093/aob/mcx145] [PMID: 29293871]

[12]   Cavalheiro CV, Rosso VD, Paulus E, *et al.* Composição química de folhas de oliveira (*Olea europaea* L.) da região de Caçapava do Sul, RS, Brazil. Ciencia Rural, Santa Maria 2014; 44: 1874-9.
[http://dx.doi.org/10.1590/0103-8478cr20131139]

[13]   Abaza L, Taamalli A, Nsir H, Zarrouk M. Olive tree (*Olea europaea* L.) leaves: importance and advances in the analysis of phenolic compounds. Antioxidants 2015; 4(4): 682-98.
[http://dx.doi.org/10.3390/antiox4040682] [PMID: 26783953]

[14]   Lawrendiadis G. Contribution to the knowledge of the medicinal plants of Greece. Planta Med 1961; 9: 164-9.
[http://dx.doi.org/10.1055/s-0028-1100338]

[15]   Ribeiro R de A, de Barros F, de Melo MM, *et al.* Acute diuretic effects in conscious rats produced by some medicinal plants used in the state of São Paulo, Brasil. J Ethnopharmacol 1988; 24(1): 19-29.
[http://dx.doi.org/10.1016/0378-8741(88)90136-5] [PMID: 3199837]

[16]   Tahraoui A, El-Hilaly J, Israili ZH, Lyoussi B. Ethnopharmacological survey of plants used in the traditional treatment of hypertension and diabetes in south-eastern Morocco (Errachidia province). J Ethnopharmacol 2007; 110(1): 105-17.
[http://dx.doi.org/10.1016/j.jep.2006.09.011] [PMID: 17052873]

[17]   Eddouks M, Maghrani M, Lemhadri A, Ouahidi ML, Jouad H. Ethnopharmacological survey of medicinal plants used for the treatment of diabetes mellitus, hypertension and cardiac diseases in the south-east region of Morocco (Tafilalet). J Ethnopharmacol 2002; 82(2-3): 97-103.
[http://dx.doi.org/10.1016/S0378-8741(02)00164-2] [PMID: 12241983]

[18]   Ali-Shtayeh MS, Jamous RM, Jamous RM. Complementary and alternative medicine use amongst Palestinian diabetic patients. Complement Ther Clin Pract 2012; 18(1): 16-21.
[http://dx.doi.org/10.1016/j.ctcp.2011.09.001] [PMID: 22196568]

[19]   Alarcon-Aguilara FJ, Roman-Ramos R, Perez-Gutierrez S, Aguilar-Contreras A, Contreras-Weber CC, Flores-Saenz JL. Study of the anti-hyperglycemic effect of plants used as antidiabetics. J Ethnopharmacol 1998; 61(2): 101-10.
[http://dx.doi.org/10.1016/S0378-8741(98)00020-8] [PMID: 9683340]

[20]   Amel B. Traditional treatment of high blood pressure and diabetes in Souk Ahras district. J Pharmacogn Phytother 2013; 5: 12-20.

[21]   Vogel P, Kasper Machado I, Garavaglia J, Zani VT, de Souza D, Morelo Dal Bosco S. Polyphenols benefits of olive leaf (*Olea europaea* L) to human health. Nutr Hosp 2014; 31(3): 1427-33.
[PMID: 25726243]

[22]   Ferreira ICFR, Barros L, Soares ME, Bastos ML, Pereira JA. Antioxidant activity and phenolic contents of *Olea europaea* L. leaves sprayed with different copper formulations. Food Chem 2007; 103: 188-95.
[http://dx.doi.org/10.1016/j.foodchem.2006.08.006]

[23]   Benavente-García O, Castillo J, Lorente J, Ortuño A, Del Río JA. Antioxidant activity of phenolics extracted from *Olea europea* L. leaves. Food Chem 2000; 68: 457-62.
[http://dx.doi.org/10.1016/S0308-8146(99)00221-6]

[24]   Silva S, Gomes L, Leitao F, Coelho AV, Vilas Boas L. Phenolic compounds and antioxidant activity of *Olea europaea* L. fruits and leaves. Food Sci Technol Int 2006; 12: 385-96.
[http://dx.doi.org/10.1177/1082013206070166]

[25]   Susalit E, Agus N, Effendi I, *et al.* Olive (*Olea europaea*) leaf extract effective in patients with stage-1 hypertension: comparison with Captopril. Phytomedicine 2011; 18(4): 251-8.
[http://dx.doi.org/10.1016/j.phymed.2010.08.016] [PMID: 21036583]

[26]   Jemai H, Bouaziz M, Fki I, El Feki A, Sayadi S. Hypolipidimic and antioxidant activities of oleuropein and its hydrolysis derivative-rich extracts from Chemlali olive leaves. Chem Biol Interact 2008; 176(2-3): 88-98.

[http://dx.doi.org/10.1016/j.cbi.2008.08.014] [PMID: 18823963]

[27]   Andreadou I, Iliodromitis EK, Mikros E, *et al.* The olive constituent oleuropein exhibits anti-ischemic, antioxidative, and hypolipidemic effects in anesthetized rabbits. J Nutr 2006; 136(8): 2213-9.
[http://dx.doi.org/10.1093/jn/136.8.2213] [PMID: 16857843]

[28]   Jemai H, El Feki A, Sayadi S. Antidiabetic and antioxidant effects of hydroxytyrosol and oleuropein from olive leaves in alloxan-diabetic rats. J Agric Food Chem 2009; 57(19): 8798-804.
[http://dx.doi.org/10.1021/jf901280r] [PMID: 19725535]

[29]   Khalatbary AR, Zarrinjoei GR. Anti-inflammatory effect of oleuropein in experimental rat spinal cord trauma. Iran Red Crescent Med J 2012; 14(4): 229-34.
[PMID: 22754686]

[30]   Giner E, Andújar I, Recio MC, Ríos JL, Cerdá-Nicolás JM, Giner RM. Oleuropein ameliorates acute colitis in mice. J Agric Food Chem 2011; 59(24): 12882-92.
[http://dx.doi.org/10.1021/jf203715m] [PMID: 22114936]

[31]   Giner E, Recio MC, Ríos JL, Giner RM. Oleuropein protects against dextran sodium sulfate-induced chronic colitis in mice. J Nat Prod 2013; 76(6): 1113-20.
[http://dx.doi.org/10.1021/np400175b] [PMID: 23758110]

[32]   Korukluoglu M, Sahan Y, Yigit A. Antifungal properties of olive leaf extracts and their phenolic compounds. J Food Saf 2008; 28: 76-87.
[http://dx.doi.org/10.1111/j.1745-4565.2007.00096.x]

[33]   Pereira AP, Ferreira ICFR, Marcelino F, *et al.* Phenolic compounds and antimicrobial activity of olive (*Olea europaea* L. Cv. Cobrançosa) leaves. Molecules 2007; 12(5): 1153-62.
[http://dx.doi.org/10.3390/12051153] [PMID: 17873849]

[34]   Kearney PM, Whelton M, Reynolds K, Whelton PK, He J. Worldwide prevalence of hypertension: a systematic review. J Hypertens 2004; 22(1): 11-9.
[http://dx.doi.org/10.1097/00004872-200401000-00003] [PMID: 15106785]

[35]   Mills KT, Bundy JD, Kelly TN, *et al.* Global disparities of hypertension prevalence and control: a systematic analysis of population-based studies from 90 countries. Circulation 2016; 134(6): 441-50.
[http://dx.doi.org/10.1161/CIRCULATIONAHA.115.018912] [PMID: 27502908]

[36]   Williams B, Mancia G, Spiering W, *et al.* 2018 ESC/ESH Guidelines for the management of arterial hypertension. Eur Heart J 2018; 39(33): 3021-104.
[http://dx.doi.org/10.1093/eurheartj/ehy339] [PMID: 30165516]

[37]   Whelton PK, Carey RM, Aronow WS, *et al.* 2017 ACC/AHA/AAPA/ABC/ACPM/AGS/APhA/ASH/ASPC/NMA/PCNA guideline for the prevention, detection, evaluation, and management of high blood pressure in adults: a report of the American College of Cardiology/American Heart Association Task Force on Clinical Practice Guidelines. Hypertension 2018; 71(6): e13-e115.
[PMID: 29133356]

[38]   Al Disi SS, Anwar MA, Eid AH. Anti-hypertensive herbs and their mechanisms of action: Part I. Front Pharmacol 2016; 6: 323.
[http://dx.doi.org/10.3389/fphar.2015.00323] [PMID: 26834637]

[39]   Anwar MA, Al Disi SS, Eid AH. Anti-hypertensive herbs and their mechanisms of action: Part II. Front Pharmacol 2016; 7: 50.
[http://dx.doi.org/10.3389/fphar.2016.00050] [PMID: 27014064]

[40]   Dernini S, Berry EM. Mediterranean diet: from a healthy diet to a sustainable dietary pattern. Front Nutr 2015; 2: 15.
[http://dx.doi.org/10.3389/fnut.2015.00015] [PMID: 26284249]

[41]   Lockyer S, Yaqoob P. Parveen, Spencer JPE, Rowland I. Olive leaf phenolics, and cardiovascular risk reduction: Physiological effects and mechanisms of action. Nutr Aging (Amst) 2012; 1: 125-40.
[http://dx.doi.org/10.3233/NUA-2012-0011]

[42]   Gorzynik-Debicka M, Przychodzen P, Cappello F, *et al.* Potential health benefits of olive oil and plant polyphenols. Int J Mol Sci 2018; 19(3)E686
[http://dx.doi.org/10.3390/ijms19030686] [PMID: 29495598]

[43]   Psaltopoulou T, Naska A, Orfanos P, Trichopoulos D, Mountokalakis T, Trichopoulou A. Olive oil, the Mediterranean diet, and arterial blood pressure: the Greek European Prospective Investigation into Cancer and Nutrition (EPIC) study. Am J Clin Nutr 2004; 80(4): 1012-8.
[http://dx.doi.org/10.1093/ajcn/80.4.1012] [PMID: 15447913]

[44]   Estruch R, Ros E, Salas-Salvadó J, *et al.* Primary prevention of cardiovascular disease with a Mediterranean diet. N Engl J Med 2013; 368(14): 1279-90.
[http://dx.doi.org/10.1056/NEJMoa1200303] [PMID: 23432189]

[45]   Cherif S, Rahal N, Haouala M, *et al.* [A clinical trial of a titrated Olea extract in the treatment of essential arterial hypertension]. J Pharm Belg 1996; 51(2): 69-71.
[PMID: 8786521]

[46]   Perrinjaquet-Moccetti T, Busjahn A, Schmidlin C, Schmidt A, Bradl B, Aydogan C. Food supplementation with an olive (*Olea europaea* L.) leaf extract reduces blood pressure in borderline hypertensive monozygotic twins. Phytother Res 2008; 22(9): 1239-42.
[http://dx.doi.org/10.1002/ptr.2455] [PMID: 18729245]

[47]   de Bock M, Derraik JG, Brennan CM, *et al.* Olive (*Olea europaea* L.) leaf polyphenols improve insulin sensitivity in middle-aged overweight men: a randomized, placebo-controlled, crossover trial. PLoS One 2013; 8(3)e57622
[http://dx.doi.org/10.1371/journal.pone.0057622] [PMID: 23516412]

[48]   Cabrera-Vique C, Navarro-Alarcón M, Rodríguez-Martínez C, Fonollá-Joya J. Efecto hipotensor de un extracto de componentes bioactivos de hojas de olivo: estudio clínico preliminar. Nutr Hosp 2015; 32: 242-9.
[PMID: 26262723]

[49]   Lockyer S, Rowland I, Spencer JPE, Yaqoob P, Stonehouse W. Impact of phenolic-rich olive leaf extract on blood pressure, plasma lipids and inflammatory markers: a randomised controlled trial. Eur J Nutr 2017; 56(4): 1421-32.
[http://dx.doi.org/10.1007/s00394-016-1188-y] [PMID: 26951205]

[50]   Javadi H, Yaghoobzadeh H, Esfahani Z, Reza Memarzadeh M, Mehdi Mirhashemi S. Effects of olive leaf extract on metabolic response, liver and kidney functions, and inflammatory biomarkers in hypertensive patients. Pak J Biol Sci 2019; 22(7): 342-8.
[http://dx.doi.org/10.3923/pjbs.2019.342.348] [PMID: 31930845]

[51]   Hansen K, Adsersen A, Christensen SB, Jensen SR, Nyman U, Smitt UW. Isolation of an angiotensin converting enzyme (ACE) inhibitor from *Olea europaea* and *Olea lancea*. Phytomedicine 1996; 2(4): 319-25.
[http://dx.doi.org/10.1016/S0944-7113(96)80076-6] [PMID: 23194770]

[52]   Gilani AH, Khan AU, Shah AJ, Connor J, Jabeen Q. Blood pressure lowering effect of olive is mediated through calcium channel blockade. Int J Food Sci Nutr 2005; 56(8): 613-20.
[http://dx.doi.org/10.1080/09637480500539420] [PMID: 16638666]

[53]   Scheffler A, Rauwald HW, Kampa B, Mann U, Mohr FW, Dhein S. *Olea europaea* leaf extract exerts L-type Ca($^{2+}$) channel antagonistic effects. J Ethnopharmacol 2008; 120(2): 233-40.
[http://dx.doi.org/10.1016/j.jep.2008.08.018] [PMID: 18790040]

[54]   Mnafgui K, Khlif I, Hajji R, *et al.* Preventive effects of oleuropein against cardiac remodeling after myocardial infarction in Wistar rat through inhibiting angiotensin-converting enzyme activity. Toxicol Mech Methods 2015; 25(7): 538-46.
[http://dx.doi.org/10.3109/15376516.2015.1053648] [PMID: 26056852]

[55]   Moreno-Luna R, Muñoz-Hernandez R, Miranda ML, *et al.* Olive oil polyphenols decrease blood

pressure and improve endothelial function in young women with mild hypertension. Am J Hypertens 2012; 25(12): 1299-304.
[http://dx.doi.org/10.1038/ajh.2012.128] [PMID: 22914255]

[56] Zarzuelo A, Duarte J, Jiménez J, González M, Utrilla MP. Vasodilator effect of olive leaf. Planta Med 1991; 57(5): 417-9.
[http://dx.doi.org/10.1055/s-2006-960138] [PMID: 1798793]

[57] Martín-Peláez S, Castañer O, Konstantinidou V, *et al.* Effect of olive oil phenolic compounds on the expression of blood pressure-related genes in healthy individuals. Eur J Nutr 2017; 56(2): 663-70.
[http://dx.doi.org/10.1007/s00394-015-1110-z] [PMID: 26658900]

[58] Klonoff DC, Schwartz DM. An economic analysis of interventions for diabetes. Diabetes Care 2000; 23(3): 390-404.
[http://dx.doi.org/10.2337/diacare.23.3.390] [PMID: 10868871]

[59] Gagliardino JJ, Martella A, Etchegoyen GS, *et al.* Hospitalization and re-hospitalization of people with and without diabetes in La Plata, Argentina: comparison of their clinical characteristics and costs. Diabetes Res Clin Pract 2004; 65(1): 51-9.
[http://dx.doi.org/10.1016/j.diabres.2003.11.011] [PMID: 15163478]

[60] Cho NH, Shaw JE, Karuranga S, *et al.* IDF Diabetes Atlas: Global estimates of diabetes prevalence for 2017 and projections for 2045. Diabetes Res Clin Pract 2018; 138: 271-81.
[http://dx.doi.org/10.1016/j.diabres.2018.02.023] [PMID: 29496507]

[61] Standards of medical care in diabetes--2014. Diabetes Care 2014; 37 (Suppl. 1): S14-80.
[http://dx.doi.org/10.2337/dc14-S014] [PMID: 24357209]

[62] Kahn SE, Prigeon RL, McCulloch DK, *et al.* Quantification of the relationship between insulin sensitivity and β-cell function in human subjects. Evidence for a hyperbolic function. Diabetes 1993; 42(11): 1663-72.
[http://dx.doi.org/10.2337/diab.42.11.1663] [PMID: 8405710]

[63] Ferrannini E, Gastaldelli A, Miyazaki Y, Matsuda M, Mari A, DeFronzo RA. β-Cell function in subjects spanning the range from normal glucose tolerance to overt diabetes: a new analysis. J Clin Endocrinol Metab 2005; 90(1): 493-500.
[http://dx.doi.org/10.1210/jc.2004-1133] [PMID: 15483086]

[64] Weyer C, Bogardus C, Mott DM, Pratley RE. The natural history of insulin secretory dysfunction and insulin resistance in the pathogenesis of type 2 diabetes mellitus. J Clin Invest 1999; 104(6): 787-94.
[http://dx.doi.org/10.1172/JCI7231] [PMID: 10491414]

[65] Butler AE, Janson J, Bonner-Weir S, Ritzel R, Rizza RA, Butler PC. β-cell deficit and increased β-cell apoptosis in humans with type 2 diabetes. Diabetes 2003; 52(1): 102-10.
[http://dx.doi.org/10.2337/diabetes.52.1.102] [PMID: 12502499]

[66] Sakuraba H, Mizukami H, Yagihashi N, Wada R, Hanyu C, Yagihashi S. Reduced β-cell mass and expression of oxidative stress-related DNA damage in the islet of Japanese Type II diabetic patients. Diabetologia 2002; 45(1): 85-96.
[http://dx.doi.org/10.1007/s125-002-8248-z] [PMID: 11845227]

[67] Araki E, Oyadomari S, Mori M. Impact of endoplasmic reticulum stress pathway on pancreatic β-cells and diabetes mellitus. Exp Biol Med (Maywood) 2003; 228(10): 1213-7.
[http://dx.doi.org/10.1177/153537020322801018] [PMID: 14610263]

[68] Tuomilehto J, Lindström J, Eriksson JG, *et al.* Prevention of type 2 diabetes mellitus by changes in lifestyle among subjects with impaired glucose tolerance. N Engl J Med 2001; 344(18): 1343-50.
[http://dx.doi.org/10.1056/NEJM200105033441801] [PMID: 11333990]

[69] Knowler WC, Barrett-Connor E, Fowler SE, *et al.* Reduction in the incidence of type 2 diabetes with lifestyle intervention or metformin. N Engl J Med 2002; 346(6): 393-403.
[http://dx.doi.org/10.1056/NEJMoa012512] [PMID: 11832527]

[70]   Chiasson JL, Josse RG, Gomis R, Hanefeld M, Karasik A, Laakso M. Acarbose for prevention of type 2 diabetes mellitus: the STOP-NIDDM randomised trial. Lancet 2002; 359(9323): 2072-7.
[http://dx.doi.org/10.1016/S0140-6736(02)08905-5] [PMID: 12086760]

[71]   Gerstein HC, Yusuf S, Bosch J, *et al.* Effect of rosiglitazone on the frequency of diabetes in patients with impaired glucose tolerance or impaired fasting glucose: a randomised controlled trial. Lancet 2006; 368(9541): 1096-105.
[http://dx.doi.org/10.1016/S0140-6736(06)69420-8] [PMID: 16997664]

[72]   Ríos JL, Francini F, Schinella GR. Natural products for the treatment of type 2 diabetes mellitus. Planta Med 2015; 81(12-13): 975-94.
[http://dx.doi.org/10.1055/s-0035-1546131] [PMID: 26132858]

[73]   El SN, Karakaya S. Olive tree (*Olea europaea*) leaves: potential beneficial effects on human health. Nutr Rev 2009; 67(11): 632-8.
[http://dx.doi.org/10.1111/j.1753-4887.2009.00248.x] [PMID: 19906250]

[74]   Cumaoğlu A, Rackova L, Stefek M, Kartal M, Maechler P, Karasu C. Effects of olive leaf polyphenols against H_2O_2 toxicity in insulin secreting β-cells. Acta Biochim Pol 2011; 58(1): 45-50.
[http://dx.doi.org/10.18388/abp.2011_2284] [PMID: 21383995]

[75]   Ben Salem M, Affes H, Ksouda K, Sahnoun Z, Mounir Zeghal K, Hammami S. Pharmacological activities of *Olea europaea* leaves. J Food Process Preserv 2015; 39: 3128-36.
[http://dx.doi.org/10.1111/jfpp.12341]

[76]   Al-Azzawie HF, Alhamdani M-SS. Hypoglycemic and antioxidant effect of oleuropein in alloxan-diabetic rabbits. Life Sci 2006; 78(12): 1371-7.
[http://dx.doi.org/10.1016/j.lfs.2005.07.029] [PMID: 16236331]

[77]   Sato H, Genet C, Strehle A, *et al.* Anti-hyperglycemic activity of a TGR5 agonist isolated from *Olea europaea*. Biochem Biophys Res Commun 2007; 362(4): 793-8.
[http://dx.doi.org/10.1016/j.bbrc.2007.06.130] [PMID: 17825251]

[78]   Eidi A, Eidi M, Darzi R. Antidiabetic effect of *Olea europaea* L. in normal and diabetic rats. Phytother Res 2009; 23(3): 347-50.
[http://dx.doi.org/10.1002/ptr.2629] [PMID: 18844257]

[79]   Dubey VK, Patil CR, Kamble SM, *et al.* Oleanolic acid prevents progression of streptozotocin induced diabetic nephropathy and protects renal microstructures in Sprague Dawley rats. J Pharmacol Pharmacother 2013; 4(1): 47-52.
[http://dx.doi.org/10.4103/0976-500X.107678] [PMID: 23662024]

[80]   Wainstein J, Ganz T, Boaz M, *et al.* Olive leaf extract as a hypoglycemic agent in both human diabetic subjects and in rats. J Med Food 2012; 15(7): 605-10.
[http://dx.doi.org/10.1089/jmf.2011.0243] [PMID: 22512698]

[81]   Bennani-Kabchi N, Fdhil H, Cherrah Y, El Bouayadi F, Kehel L, Marquie G. Effet thérapeutique des feuilles d'*Olea europea* var. *oleaster* sur le métabolisme glucido-lipidique chez le rat des sables (*Psammomys obesus*) obèse prédiabétique. Ann Pharm Fr 2000; 58(4): 271-7.
[PMID: 10915976]

[82]   Guex CG, Reginato FZ, de Jesus PR, Brondani JC, Lopes GHH, Bauermann LF. Antidiabetic effects of *Olea europaea* L. leaves in diabetic rats induced by high-fat diet and low-dose streptozotocin. J Ethnopharmacol 2019; 235: 1-7.
[http://dx.doi.org/10.1016/j.jep.2019.02.001] [PMID: 30721736]

[83]   Hasani-Ranjbar S, Nayebi N, Moradi L, Mehri A, Larijani B, Abdollahi M. The efficacy and safety of herbal medicines used in the treatment of hyperlipidemia; a systematic review. Curr Pharm Des 2010; 16(26): 2935-47.
[http://dx.doi.org/10.2174/138161210793176464] [PMID: 20858178]

[84]   Léger CL, Carbonneau MA, Michel F, *et al.* A thromboxane effect of a hydroxytyrosol-rich olive oil

wastewater extract in patients with uncomplicated type I diabetes. Eur J Clin Nutr 2005; 59(5): 727-30.
[http://dx.doi.org/10.1038/sj.ejcn.1602133] [PMID: 15798774]

[85]　Florentin M, Liberopoulos E, Elisaf MS, Tsimihodimos V. No effect of fenugreek, bergamot and olive leaf extract on glucose homeostasis in patients with prediabetes: a randomized double-blind placebo-controlled study. Arch Med Sci Atheroscler Dis 2019; 4: e162-6.
[http://dx.doi.org/10.5114/amsad.2019.86756] [PMID: 31448348]

[86]　Pyner A, Chan SY, Tumova S, Kerimi A, Williamson G. Indirect chronic effects of an oleuropein-rich olive leaf extract on sucrase-isomaltase*in vitro* and *in vivo*. Nutrients 2019; 11(7)E1505
[http://dx.doi.org/10.3390/nu11071505] [PMID: 31266155]

[87]　Acar-Tek N, Ağagündüz D. Olive leaf (*Olea europaea* L. folium): Potential effects on glycemia and lipidemia. Ann Nutr Metab 2020; 76(1): 10-5.
[http://dx.doi.org/10.1159/000505508] [PMID: 31901903]

CHAPTER 4

Medicinal Plants from Genus *Costus* in the Management of Diabetes

Ankit P. Laddha[1], **Kaveri M. Adki**[1], **Manisha J. Oza**[1,2], **Anil Bhanudas Gaikwad**[3] and **Yogesh A. Kulkarni**[1,*]

[1] *Shobhaben Pratapbhai Patel School of Pharmacy & Technology Management, SVKM's NMIMS, V.L. Mehta Road, Vile Parle (West), Mumbai-400056, India*

[2] *SVKM's Dr. Bhanuben Nanavati College of Pharmacy, V.L. Mehta Road, Vile Parle (West), Mumbai-400056, India*

[3] *Department of Pharmacy, Birla Institute of Technology and Science, Pilani, Pilani Campus Pilani- 333031, Rajasthan, India*

Abstract: Diabetes is a chronic metabolic disorder characterized by a persistent increased level of glucose in the blood. The uncontrolled glucose level in the blood is associated with a defect in insulin secretion, insulin action, or both, which leads to the progression of oxidative stress. It also affects metabolic, genetic, and haemodynamic systems by activating the polyol pathway, protein kinase C pathway, and hexosamine pathway. According to the World Health Organization (WHO) report, globally, an estimated 422 million adults were living with diabetes in 2014, compared to 108 million in 1980.

Various medicinal plants, as well as phytochemicals like alkaloids, glycosides, terpenes, and polyphenols, have been thoroughly studied for their activity in the management of diabetes. Recent data showed that around 1200 traditional plants have been used for real or perceived benefit in the treatment of diabetes. *Costus* (Linn.) is an important genus belonging to the family '*Costaceae*' containing approximately 200 species. The plants have spirally arranged leaves and rhizomes being free from aromatic essential oils and tropically distributed in nature. In Ayurveda, the rhizomes of plants are described to be astringent, acrid, cooling, aphrodisiac, purgative, anthelmintic, depurative, and expectorant. Aerial parts of the plants and rhizomes are an edible and good source of carbohydrate, starch, amylase, proteins, and lipids. Recent literature shows that many species of *Costus* like *Costus pictus*, *Costus afer*, *Costus spirali*, *Costus speciosus*, and *Costus igneus* possess a significant glucose-lowering capacity. They are commonly known as 'insulin plants'. The chapter provides scientific information on plants from *genus Costus* focusing on phytochemistry, pharmacological effects specifically in diabetic conditions.

---

* **Corresponding author Yogesh A. Kulkarni:** Shobhaben Pratapbhai Patel School of Pharmacy & Technology Management, SVKM's NMIMS, V.L. Mehta Road, Vile Parle (West), Mumbai-400056, India; Tel: 91 22 42332000; E-mail: yogeshkulkarni101@yahoo.com

Mohamed Eddouks (Ed.)

Keywords: Diabetes, Genus-*Costus*, Hyperglycemia, Insulin plants, Medicinal plant, Traditional medicine.

INTRODUCTION

In many countries, traditional plant-based medicines are considered as an important part of health care. Many regions of Asia, Africa, and Central and South America have literature on traditional medicines, which is freely available and assessable by the people. In many countries like China, India, Europe, and Germany, traditional medicines are being integrated through regulation into the human healthcare system [1]. According to a report by the World Health Organization (WHO), the estimated annual global market of herbal medicine in the year 2003 was around $60 billion and by 2012, the global industry in traditional and complementary medicine (TCM) alone was reported to be worth of $83 billion. Based on the current information of the year 2019, 170 countries have confirmed their use of traditional and complementary medicine. These are the countries which have developed law, policies, rules, regulations, and offices for TCM [2].

Nowadays, healthcare systems around the world are facing major issues related to chronic illness, population aging, and healthcare cost. Traditional medicines are often seen as more accessible, more affordable, and more acceptable to local populations and can, therefore, be a tool for achieving universal health coverage [3]. 80% of people worldwide believe in herbal medicine for their primary healthcare. According to the WHO data, around 21,000 plant species are reported to have medicinal properties and around three-quarters of the world population utilizes medicinal plants and their extracts for treating various diseases [4].

Diabetes mellitus is a chronic metabolic disorder associated with the prolonged increased level of glucose in the blood [5]. Long term increased level of glucose in blood results in vascular changes and dysfunctions which are the main reasons behind mortality and morbidity among diabetic patients. Diabetes mellitus has a high prevalence rate throughout the world [6]. According to a recent statistic by the International Diabetic Federation 2017, four out of five people live with diabetes in low and middle-income countries. 425 million people have been reported to have diabetes till the year in 2017 in the world and it has been predicted that it will reach to 629 million by the year 2045 [7].

An uncontrolled level of glucose in the blood is because of abnormality in insulin secretion or insulin action. Abnormality in insulin secretion because of damaged β-cells of the pancreas is linked to the development of type-I diabetes, whereas, resistance to secreted insulin is associated with the development of type -II diabetes. Prolong uncontrolled hyperglycemia in both cases leads to the formation of reactive oxygen species by activation of the polyol pathway, protein kinase C pathway, and hexosamine pathway. It also increases advanced glycation end products (AGEs) formation. Various vital organs like kidney, eye, nerve, and heart are affected by prolonged increased blood glucose level [8 - 11].

There is an unmet need for the treatment of diabetes due to high prevalence, rapid growth rate, variable pathogenesis, and development of complications. Various treatment options like insulin therapy, blood sugar monitoring, diet therapy, and pharmacotherapy are available for diabetes [12]. Blood glucose-lowering agents like sulfonylurea or meglitinides work by stimulating insulin secretion from β cells of pancreas and drugs like biguanides and thiazolidinediones increase peripheral absorption of glucose [13]. Delay in intestinal carbohydrate absorption by α-glucosidase and reduction in hepatic gluconeogenesis by biguanides (Metformin) are another therapeutic approach for the treatment of diabetes [14]. Besides all the therapeutic benefits, these treatments are associated with some disadvantages like drug resistance, hypoglycemia, side effects, and toxicity. Drugs like sulfonylurea develop resistance in 44% of people after 6 years of treatment and many anti-diabetic drugs are withdrawn from the market because of drug-drug interactions [15]. To minimize the adverse effect of anti-diabetic drugs, many people nowadays use plant-based medicinal therapy for the management of diabetes. Plants contain various constituents like alkaloids, glycosides, polyphenols, tannins, flavonoids, and terpenoids which are reported for their anti-diabetic property [16 - 18]. Plant-based medicines act as insulinomimetic or secretagogues by restoring the function of β-pancreatic cells or inhibiting intestinal absorption of glucose. More than 400 plant species are available in the literature that possess anti-hyperglycemic activity [19].

Costaceae family of order Zingiberales is reported for its medicinal value worldwide and is commonly known as Spiral ginger. *Monocostus, Dimerocostus, Chamaecostus, Costus, Paracostus, Cheilocostus,* and *Tapeinochilos* are various genera of the Costaceae family out of which *Costus* is the largest genus which contains more than 175 species [20]. Plants from this genus are mostly found in the tropical and sub-tropical regions of Asia, Africa, and America. China, Malaysia, New Guinea, Taiwan, and India are some countries where genus *Costus*are is found in hilly regions. Detailed scientific studies have also been carried out on various species of *Costus* for its use in the treatment of cough, inflammation, rheumatism, arthritis, and diabetes. Besides this, they have also been used as anti-bacterial, anti-viral, hypolipidemic, diuretic, laxative, and purgative (Fig. 1) [21]. Some important phytoconstituents present in genus *Costus* plants responsible for pharmacological activities are mentioned in Table **1**. In addition, genus *Costus* has potent anti-diabetic properties. Eight species of genus *Costus* have been studied in detail for the antidiabetic potential. This chapter focuses on details of genus *Costus* and its phytochemistry and pharmacological effects on diabetes.

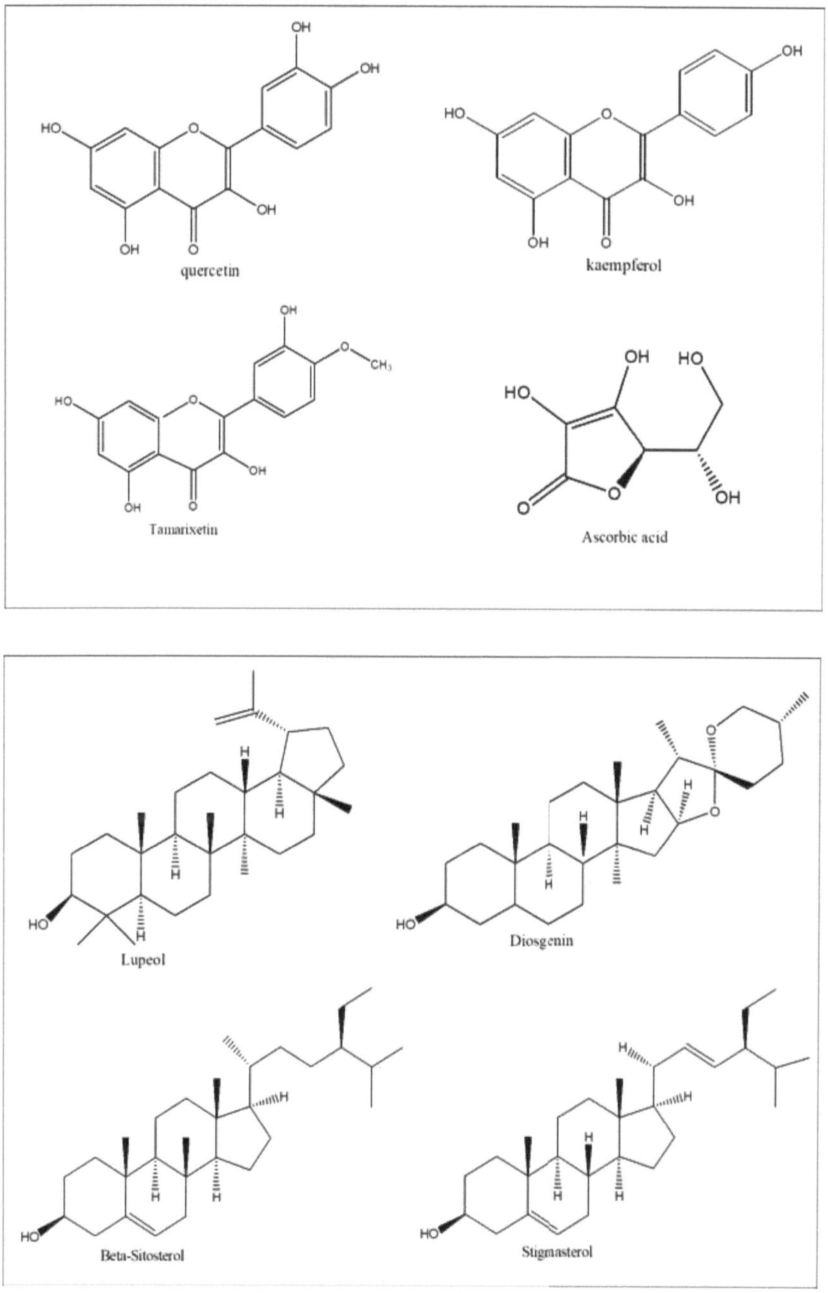

Fig. 1 cont.....

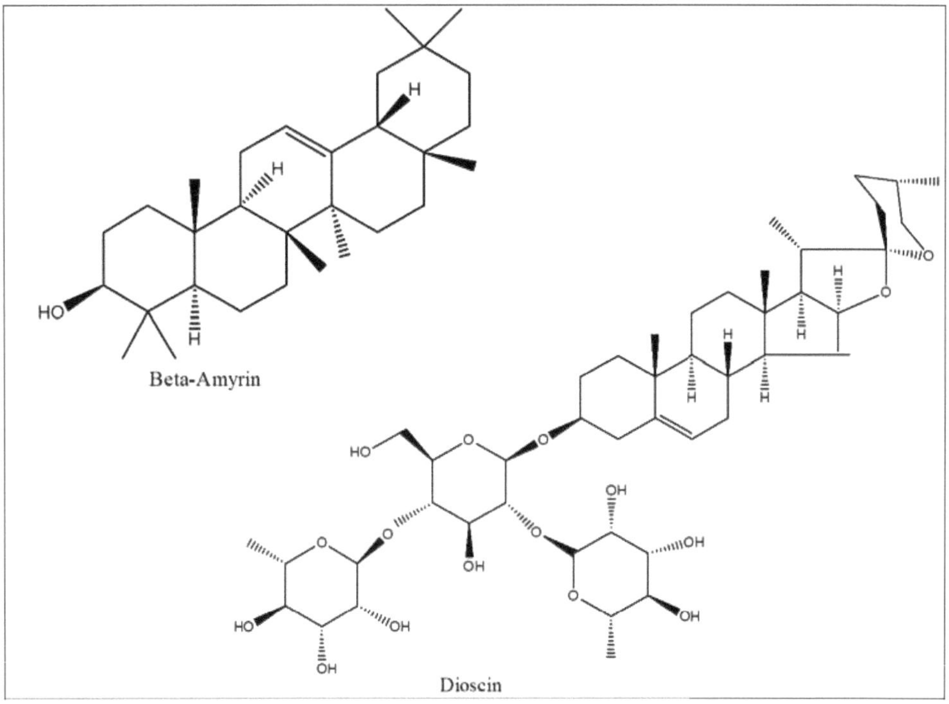

Fig. (1). Important phytoconstituents present in genus *Costus* responsible for anti-diabetic activity.

Table 1. Important species of *Costus* and their reported activities.

S. No.	Species	Plant Part Used	Pharmacological Effect	Reference
1.	*Costus afer*	Leaves	• Anti-diabetic • Anti-hyperlipidemic	[22]
2.	*Costus igneus*	Leaves	• Anti-diabetic	[23]
3.	*Costus lucanusianus*	Leaves	• Uterine relaxant activity	[24]
4.	*Costus picatus*	Leaves Stem Root	• Anti-diabetic • Anti-oxidant • Anti-microbial • Anti-cancer • Anti-fertility • Anti-helminthic • Anti-inflammatory	[25]

(Table 1) cont.....

S. No.	Species	Plant Part Used	Pharmacological Effect	Reference
5.	*Costus spectabilis*	Leaves	**In the treatment of** • Cough • Inflammation • Arthritis **Used as** • Laxative • Purgative • Diuretic • Rheumatism	[26]
6.	*Costus schlechteri*	Leaves	• Anti-diabetic	
7.	*Costus spiralis*	Leaves	**In the treatment of** • Urinary infection • Urine stone • Myocardial contractility	[27]
8.	*Costus specious*	Rhizome Stem Leaves	• Anti-diabetic • Antioxidant • Anticancer • Anti-inflammatory • Hypolipidemic • Hepatoprotective • Steroidogenic • Adaptogenic • Antimicrobial	[28]

GEOGRAPHICAL AND BOTANICAL DESCRIPTION OF GENUS *COSTUS*

All seven genera of the Costaceae family are widely spread in various parts of the world. The largest genus *Costus* is mostly indigenous to West Indies, Mexico, and some neo-tropical regions of South America. Out of its 175 species, around 20 species are found in Asia and Africa and 7 species of *Chamaecostus* genus are localized to some regions of South America. Two species each of *Paracostus* and *Dimerocostus* genus are distributed in Africa and the Central to South America region, respectively. Sixteen species of *Tapeinochilos* genus and four species of *Cheilocostus* genus are grown in Africa and Central and South America, respectively. *Monocostus* genus was found to be grown in the South American country of Peru [29].

Botanically, Genus *Costus* shows the presence of perennial herbaceous flowering plants having a long fleshy stem and edible tuberous rootstock. The plant is up to 2 feet tall, leaves are evergreen, spiral with silky pubescent base, and 4 to 8 inches in length. Flowers are terminal and densely arranged. The calyx is a funnel-shaped short tube and stamens are broad ablonged filaments. Overy is generally three celled with filiform style and semilunar stigma. Ovules are superposed and multiple in number and seeds are oval and subglobose [30].

All the species of the genus *Costus* prefer partial sunny and partial shade with a hot climatic condition for their proper growth. The plants also need moisture, fertile soil and are often grown near water.

PHYTOCHEMISTRY OF GENUS *COSTUS*

Genus *Costus* is rich in many active constituents. Different classes of phytochemicals present in genus *Costus* are classified into flavonoids and flavonoid glycoside, terpenoids, sterols, fatty acids, and steroidal saponins. Details of phytochemicals present in various species of *Costus* are presented in Table **2**.

Genus *Costus* and Diabetes

Various plant species of genus *Costus* gained much research interest for the last few years because of their reported health benefits in different traditional systems of medicine. In ancient times, genus *Costus* was used in the treatment of cough, post-partum bleeding, insufficient uterine contractility, skin diseases, snake bite, etc [34]. In recent years, many researchers have worked on the anti-diabetic activity of genus *Costus*.

Plants like *Costus pictus, Costus afer, Costus spirali, Costus speciosus,* and *Costus igneus* are scientifically studied for their role in diabetes.

Costus pictus and Diabetes

Costus pictus is popular for its name the 'insulin plant' because of its increase in insulin secretory effect. Aqueous extract of leaves of *Costus pictus* at the dose of 2 g/kg for 28 days in streptozotocin(STZ)-induced diabetic rats showed a marked reduction in the level of fasting blood glucose and a remarkable increase in serum insulin level. Besides this, aqueous extract treatment further improved diabetic condition in rats by a significant reduction in serum parameters like aspartate aminotransferase (AST), alanine aminotransferase (ALT), lipids, triglycerides, total cholesterol, urea, and albumin, which indicates its effect in preventing β-pancreatic cell damage by STZ [35]. Another study carried out on the methanolic extract of leaves of *Costus pictus* on alloxan-induced diabetes in rats showed a significant reduction in blood glucose level and lipid parameters. It also significantly increased the plasma insulin level. Besides this, the study also confirmed a regenerative effect on the pancreas, liver, and kidney after alloxan administration [36].

Table 2. Phytochemistry of *genus Costus.*

S. No.	Species	Plant part	Phytoconstituents	References
1	*Costus pictus*	Leaves	• Quercetin • Quercetin 3-*O*-neohesperidoside • Kaempferol • Kaempferol-3-0-neohesperidoside • Kaempferide-3-0 neohesperidoside • Kaempferol 3-O-α-L-rharnnopyranoside • Tamarixetin • Tamarixetin 3-O-neohesperidoside • Isorhamnetin 3-O neohesperidoside	[31]
		Stem	• Hexadecanoic acid • 9,12-octadecadienoic acid • Linalylpropanoate • Dodecanoic acid • Tetradecanoic acid • α-eudesmol • γ- -eudesmol • 4-ethoxy phenol	
		Rhizomes	• Hexadecanoic acid • Dodecanoic acid • Tetradecanoic acid • Linalool • 9, 12- octadecadienoic acid • α-terpineol	
2	*Costus speciosus*	Stem Leaves Flower	• Diosgenin	[30]
		Seeds	• Costusosides I and J • 3-O-[β-D-glucopyranosyl(1→4)-β-D-glucopyranosyl]-26-O-(β-Dglucopyranosyl-22αmethoxy (25R) furost-5-en-3β,26-diol • β-sitosterol-β-D-glucoside • Prosapogenins A and B of dioscin, dioscin, gracillin, • 3-O-[α-L-rhamnopyranosyl(1→2)-β-D-glucopyranosyl]-26-O- [β-D-glucopyranosyl]- 22α-methoxy-(25R) furost-5-en-3β,26-diol, • Protodioscin and Methyl protodioscin • Methyl hexadecanoate • Methyl octadecanoate • Tetracosanyloctadecanoate • G2-tocopherol • Diosgenin, • Glucose, • Galactose • Rhamnose	
		Roots	• 24-hydroxytriacontan-26-one • 24- hydroxytriacontan-27-one • Methyl triacontanoate • Diosgenin • Sitosterol • β-sitosterol-β-D-glucoside • Prosapogenins A and B of dioscin, dioscin, gracillin	
		Rhizomes	• Tetradecyl 13-methylpentadecanoate, • Tetra 11-methyltriadecanoate, 4- oxotriaconsanoic acid, • 14 – oxoheptacosanoic acid • 15-oxooctacosnoic acid • 28 Methyl 3-(4-hydroxyphenyl)-2Epropenoate • Diosgenin • Dioscin • Gracillin • β-sitosterol-β -D-glucoside	
3	*Costus spicatus*	Leaves	• Tamarixetin 3-O-neohesperidoside • Kaempferide 3-O-neohesperidoside • Quercetin 3-Oneohesperidoside	[32]

(Table 2) cont.....

S. No.	Species	Plant part	Phytoconstituents	References
4	*Costus afer*	Leaves	• Oxo-sterol derivative • β-sitosterol • Linoleic acid • Sigmasterol	[33]
		Roots	• Aferosides B and C • Dioscin • Paryphyllin C	
		Stem	• Palmitic acid • Oleic acid • Linoleic acid • Stearic acid • Myristic acid • Lauric acids • Arachidic acid • Succinic acid	
5	*Costus ingneus*	Seed	• Dioscin, • Prosapogenis – A, and – B of dioscin • Protodioscin • Methyl protodioscin • Gracillin • Costusoside • β-sitosterol	[33]
		Leaves	• Tigogenin • Gracillin • Sitosterol • D-Glocoside	
		Rhizomes	• Diosgenin, • Prosapoenin B of dioscin, • Diosgenone, • Cycloartanol, 25-encycloartenol • Octacosanoic acid	

In vivo and *in vitro* studies carried out by Gireesh and co-workers revealed that aqueous extract of *Costus pictus* leaves showed a significantly decreased level of blood glucose and significantly increased the level of insulin in diabetic rats. The *in vitro* study carried out with pancreatic islet culture showed significant increase glucose-induced insulin secretion at both 4 mM and 20 mM glucose concentrations after *Costus pictus* leaves extract treatment which indicates release and utilization of glucose from the pancreatic cells [37].

Costus pictus plant is also reported to have anti-oxidant activity because of the presence of polyphenolic phytoconstituents. Methanolic extract of leaves and rhizomes of *Costu spictus* showed anti-oxidant activity which is 89.5 to 90% as that of standard butylated hydroxyl toluene (BHT) at concentration 400 μg/mL [38]. Another *in vitro* study carried out on aqueous, methanolic, ethanolic, and ethyl acetate extracts of *Costus pictus* showed significant inhibitory activity on carbohydrate hydrolyzing enzyme. α-amylase and α-glucosidase inhibition are linked with its anti-diabetic activity [39]. The aqueous extract showed a direct stimulatory effect on insulin secretion in MIN6 β-cell line and isolated mouse and human islets. The effect was attributed to increased Ca^{2+} levels through voltage-gated ion channel in β-cell because of *Costus pictus* aqueous extract treatment [40].

Costus afer and Diabetes

Costus afer is also reported for its anti-diabetic potential. Aqueous extract of *Costus afer* leaves at a dose of 375, 750, and 1125 mg/kg in alloxan-induced diabetic rats prevented pancreatic tissue damage and showed the anti-diabetic property. Effect of *Costus afer* is observed because of the presence of active phytoconstituents like glycosides, tannins, saponins, terpenoids, flavonoids, and alkaloids [41]. *Costus afer* is also reported for its anti-oxidant potential. A recent study by Tchamgoue and co-workers reported that treatment of STZ intoxicated rats with hydroalcoholic extract of *Costes afer* leaves at the doses of 250, 500, and 1000 mg/kg prevented cardiac, hepatic, and renal tissues from oxidative damage. Besides, this treatment also maintained the level of biochemical parameters and lipid markers [42].

In vitro study showed that methanolic extract of *Costus afer* leaves inhibited intestinal glucose uptake. Results confirmed that the methanolic extract of the leaf has more effect than that of methanolic extract of the stem and rhizome [43]. Toxicity and anti-diabetic study reported by Barminas and co-workers showed that methanolic extract of leaf of *Costus afer* is safe at 5000 mg/kg oral dose and showed beneficial anti-diabetic activity at the doses of 100 and 300 mg/kg after 21 days treatment [44]. *Costus afer* rhizome is also effective in diabetes. *In vitro* study was carried out on ethyl acetate extract of rhizome and methanol leaf extracts possess α-amylase and α-glucosidase inhibitory activity having IC_{50} of 0.10 and 5.99 mg/mL, respectively. In addition to this, hexane extract showed the high anti-oxidant property. The presence of alkaloids, flavonoids, phenols, and tannins is responsible for anti-oxidant and carbohydrate hydrolyzing enzyme inhibitory activity [22]. Crude juice stem of *Costus afer* possesses potent anti-diabetic effect. Alloxan-induced diabetic animals administered with 1.5 ml of fresh crude stem juice of *Costus afer* for 14 days showed a significant effect in diabetes by reducing blood glucose level. It also helped in improving hematological parameters in diabetic condition [45].

Aqueous stem extract of *Costus afer* at doses of 500, 1000, and 1500 mg/kg and in combination with metformin at low dose showed a significant reduction in blood sugar and β pancreatic cell regeneration in STZ-induced diabetic rats [46]. Aqueous stem extract was also been studied at 1, 2, and 3 g/kg dose in alloxan-induced diabetes. Liver marker enzyme and pancreatic cells were restored at all dose levels [47].

Costus speciosus and Diabetes

Costus specious is a well-known plant species for its anti-oxidant and anti-diabetic properties. Various phytoconstituents present in *Costus specious* species are scientifically proven for their anti-oxidant and anti-diabetic potential. Eremanthin isolated form *Costus specious* possesses strong anti-diabetic properties. Administration of eremanthin to STZ-induced diabetic rats at the dose of 20 mg/kg for 60 days significantly improved plasma insulin, tissue glycogen, HDL-cholesterol, and serum protein level. In addition to this, Ermanthin treatment significantly reduced glycosylated haemoglobin level and elevated serum lipid markers [48]. Costunolide and eremanthin isolated from *Costus specious* rhizome prevented brain, liver, heart, kidney, and pancreas damage because of their anti-oxidant potential [49]. *Costus specious* rhizome has also been studied for its anti-diabetic potential. Methanolic extract of rhizome at the dose of 200 mg/kg for 14 days reduced blood glucose level and improved lipid profile [50]. A study by Revathy and co-workers also confirmed that rhizome extract (200 mg/kg) improved liver glycogen, insulin, and lactate dehydrogenase level which helps in peripheral utilization of glucose. This treatment also maintains biochemical parameters levels like AST, ALT, albumin, creatinine, blood urea nitrogen and increases total protein level [51]. *Costus specious* plant has also been studied at the molecular level for its anti-diabetic property. Various enzymes like glucokinase, aldolase, pyruvate kinase, succinate dehydrogenase, and glycogen synthase play an important role in hepatic glucose uptake and insulin secretion from pancreatic β-cells. Glycogenesis is a pathway for glucose utilization, which is affected in diabetic rats because of decreased levels of glycogen synthase. Treatment of diabetic rats with *Costus specious* root extract at a dose of 400 and 600 mg/kg significantly improved the level of glycogen synthase after 4 weeks of treatment [52]. Aqueous and alcoholic extracts of leaves of *Costus specious* at the doses of 500 and 1500 mg/kg improved high fat induced type-II diabetes by reversing high-fat diet-induced insulin resistance [53]. Diosgenin, an important phytoconstituent present in *Costus specious,* was also reported for its glucose-lowering activity [54]. A formulation based study of *Costus specious* was also carried out. Poly-lactic-coglycolic acid (PLGA) encapsulation nanoformulation of ethanolic extract of *Costus specious* suppressed transcription of the gene involved in pancreatic insulin and hepatic glucose production. Nanoformulation also stimulated the expression of GLUT-4 in the muscle of STZ-induced diabetic rats. In addition to this, nanoformulation of *Costus specious* decreased abnormal level of lipid markers and reduced elevated levels of AST, ALT, lactate dehydrogenase (LDH), alkaline phosphatase (ALP), and acid phosphatase towards normal [55].

Costus igneus and Diabetes

Costus igneus is rich in carbohydrates, proteins, triterpenoids, alkaloids, tannins, saponins, flavonoids, and steroids. Thin-layer chromatography and high-performance liquid chromatography studies were carried out to confirm the presence of quercetin in *Costus igneus* which is responsible for its anti-diabetic potential. Computational study showed that quercetin has a binding energy of 7.28 kcal/mol with insulin receptor tyrosine kinase which is enough for binding to the receptor responsible for anti-diabetic effect [56]. Dexamethasone, a corticosteroid administration, is associated with hyperglycemia condition. Aqueous extract of *Costus igneus* at the doses of 100, 250, and 500 mg/kg to dexamethasone administered rat significantly reduced the fasting and postprandial blood sugar levels and reduced it to normal after 9 days for treatment [57]. Ethanolic extract of leaves of *Costus ignus* showed the presence of alkaloids and steroids. Alloxan-induced diabetic rats administered with ethanolic extract of *Costus ignus* leaves (500 mg/kg) for 14 days showed potent anti-diabetic activity with high glucose tolerance ability [58]. *Costus ignus* was also reported for its protective effect in the pre-diabetic stage. Pre-treatment and post-treatment of the isolated fraction of petroleum ether extract of *Costus igneus* to neonatal-streptozotocin-induced type-II diabetic rats showed a marked reduction in glucose. The effect is because of the increase in the peripheral utilization of glucose and the insulin-mimetic effect of *Costus igneus* [59]. *Costus igneus* leaf ethanolic extract synergistically reduced serum lipid levels and restored insulin and haemoglobin level at the doses of 200 and 300 mg/kg after 28 days of treatment [60].

Costus spiralis and Diabetes

Costus spiralis is reported to have 3-O-arabinoside of quercetin, guaijaverin. A recent study by Duarte and co-workers showed that acute treatment of *Costus spiralis* methanolic extract of leaves and isolated guaijaverin lowered glycemia, inhibited lipid peroxidation, and improved oral glucose tolerance in STZ-induced diabetic rats. In addition to this, it also improved lipid profile and biochemical parameters like total protein, AST, and ALT levels [61]. *In vitro* study was carried out for the determination of the α-glycosidase inhibitory activity of *Costus spiralis*. Ethyl acetate extract of leaves of *Costus spiralis* showed 1.95, 2.34, and 2.22 fold higher α-glycosidase inhibitory activity than those of acarbose and its active phytoconstituents schaftoside and isoschaftoside [62].

Details of reported anti-diabetic activities of genus *Costus* are shown in Table **3**.

Table 3. Antidiabetic studies of *genus Costus*.

S. No.	Plant Species	Plant Part and Extract Used in the Study	Dose	Animal Model Used	Duration of Study	Reference
1	*Costus pictus*	Aqueous extract of leaves	2 g/kg, *p.o*	Streptozotocin- induced diabetes	28 days	[35]
2		Methanolic extract of leaves	120 mg/kg, *p.o*	Alloxan-induced diabetes	21 days	[36]
3		Aqueous extract of leaves	250 mg/kg, *p.o*	Streptozotocin- induced diabetes	14 days	[37]
4	*Costus afer*	Aqueous extract of leaves	375, 750, and 1125 mg/kg, *p.o*	Alloxan-induced diabetes	21 days	[41]
5		Hydroalcoholic extract leaves	250, 500, and 1000 mg/kg, *p.o*	Streptozotocin- induced diabetes	60 days	[42]
6		Stem Juice	1.5 ml	Alloxan-induced diabetes	14 days	[45]
8		Aqueous stem extract	500, 1000 and 1500 mg/kg, *p.o*	Streptozotocin-induced diabetes	3, 6 and 9 weeks	[46]
9		Aqueous stem extract	1,2 and 3 g/kg, *p.o*	Alloxan-induced diabetes	21 days	[47]
10		Methanolic extract of leaves	100 and 300 mg/kg, *p.o*	Alloxan-induced diabetes	21 days	[44]
11	*Costus specious*	Ethanolic extract of root	400 and 600 mg/kg, *p.o*	Streptozotocin- induced diabetes	4 weeks	[52]
12		Methanolic extract of rhizome	200 mg/kg thrice daily, *p.o*	Streptozotocin- induced diabetes	14 days	[50]
13		Aqueous and alcoholic extracts of leaves	500 and 1500 mg/kg, *p.o*	High fat diet	4 weeks	[53]
		Ethanolic extract of rhizome extract	200 mg/kg, *p.o*	Alloxan-induced diabetes	14 days	[51]

(Table 3 cont.....

S. No.	Plant Species	Plant Part and Extract Used in the Study	Dose	Animal Model Used	Duration of Study	Reference
14	*Costus igneus*	Ethanolic extract of leaves	500 mg/kg, *p.o*	Alloxan-induced diabetes	14 days	[58]
15		An isolated fraction of petroleum ether extract	20 and 40 mg/kg, *p.o*	Streptozotocin-induced diabetes neonatal rats	4th week after STZ administration and after 12th week in non-treated rats till 21 days	[59]
16		Ethanolic extract of leaves	200 and 400 mg/kg, *p.o*	Streptozotocin- induced diabetes	28 days	[60]
17		Ethanolic extract of rhizome	100 and 200 mg/kg, *p.o*	Streptozotocin-induced diabetes	30 days	[63]
18	*Costus spiralis*	Methanolic extract of leaves	250 and 500 mg/kg	Streptozotocin-induced diabetes	Single-dose study	[61]

CONCLUDING REMARKS

Diabetes mellitus is a chronic metabolic disorder associated with a persistent increased level of glucose in the blood and likely a reason behind the high rate of mortality worldwide.

Plant-based medicines received tremendous interest from researchers and medicinal practitioners over the last few years because of their various health benefits, toxicity, safety, preventive, and rejuvenating effect. Various scientific reports showed beneficial effects of genus *Costus* in the management of diabetes. In traditional literature, plants from genus *Costus* are known as 'insulin plants' because of their insulin potentiating effect. In addition to this, plants from genus *Costus* also possess strong anti-oxidant, glucose-lowering property. This medicinal value of genus *Costus* is because of the presence of phytoconstituents like flavonoids, alkaloids, tannins, saponins, and terpenes in various plant parts. Though few systematic studies have been reported with respect to antidiabetic effects of *Costus* plants, there is a need to study various phytoconstituents responsible for the therapeutic effect in diabetic conditions. Systematic clinical studies, as well as formulation development and standardization, are needed for *Costus* plants.

CONSENT FOR PUBLICATION

Not applicable.

CONFLICT OF INTEREST

There is no conflict of interest declared.

ACKNOWLEDGEMENT

Declared none.

REFERENCES

[1]   Allkin B. Useful Plants – Medicines: At Least 28,187 Plant Species are Currently Recorded as Being of Medicinal Use. Kew: Royal Botanic Gardens 2017.http://www.ncbi.nlm.nih.gov/pubmed/29144713

[2]   WHO Global Report On Traditional And Complementary Medicine 2019 http://apps.who.int/bookorders2019.

[3]   De Sousa IMC, Tesser CD, do Nascimento MC, *et al.* Traditional and complementary medicine in primary health care in Brazil. Adv Integr Med 2019; 6: S11.
[http://dx.doi.org/10.1016/j.aimed.2019.03.031]

[4]   Khan MA. Introduction and Importance of Medicinal Plants and Herbs | National Health Portal of India. https://www.nhp.gov.in/introduction-and-importance-of-medicinal-plants-and-herbs_mtl2015 [accessed 15 August 2019];

[5]   Hameed I, Masoodi SR, Mir SA, Nabi M, Ghazanfar K, Ganai BA. Type 2 diabetes mellitus: From a metabolic disorder to an inflammatory condition. World J Diabetes 2015; 6(4): 598-612.
[http://dx.doi.org/10.4239/wjd.v6.i4.598] [PMID: 25987957]

[6]   Kitada M, Ogura Y, Koya D. Rodent models of diabetic nephropathy: their utility and limitations. Int J Nephrol Renovasc Dis 2016; 9: 279-90.
[http://dx.doi.org/10.2147/IJNRD.S103784] [PMID: 27881924]

[7]   International Diabetes Federation - Facts & figures 2019; 1. https://www.idf.org/aboutdiabetes/what-is-diabetes/facts-figures.html

[8]   Kulkarni YA, Garud MS, Oza MJ, *et al.* Diabetes, diabetic complications, and flavonoids.Fruits, Vegetables, and Herbs: Bioactive Foods in Health Promotion. 77-104.

[9]   Garud MS, Kulkarni YA. Eugenol ameliorates renal damage in streptozotocin-induced diabetic rats. Flavour Fragrance J 2017; 32: 54-62.
[http://dx.doi.org/10.1002/ffj.3357]

[10]   Laddha AP, Kulkarni YA. Tannins and vascular complications of Diabetes: An update. Phytomedicine 2019; 56: 229-45.
[http://dx.doi.org/10.1016/j.phymed.2018.10.026] [PMID: 30668344]

[11]   Suryavanshi SV, Kulkarni YA. NF-κβ: A Potential Target in the Management of Vascular Complications of Diabetes. Front Pharmacol 2017; 8: 798.
[http://dx.doi.org/10.3389/fphar.2017.00798] [PMID: 29163178]

[12]   Nathan DM. Initial management of blood glucose in adults with type 2 diabet http://www.uptodate.com.proxy.medlib.uits.iu.edu/contents/initi2016.

[13]   Lorenzati B, Zucco C, Miglietta S, Lamberti F, Bruno G. Oral hypoglycemic drugs: Pathophysiological basis of their mechanism of action. Pharmaceuticals (Basel) 2010; 3(9): 3005-20.
[http://dx.doi.org/10.3390/ph3093005] [PMID: 27713388]

[14]   Kim DJ, Kang YH, Kim KK, Kim TW, Park JB, Choe M. Increased glucose metabolism and alpha-glucosidase inhibition in *Cordyceps militaris* water extract-treated HepG2 cells. Nutr Res Pract 2017; 11(3): 180-9.
[http://dx.doi.org/10.4162/nrp.2017.11.3.180] [PMID: 28584574]

[15]   Kalra S, Bahendeka S, Sahay R, *et al.* Consensus recommendations on sulfonylurea and sulfonylurea combinations in the management of Type 2 diabetes mellitus - International Task Force. Indian J Endocrinol Metab 2018; 22(1): 132-57.
[http://dx.doi.org/10.4103/ijem.IJEM_556_17] [PMID: 29535952]

[16]   Christodoulou M-I, Tchoumtchoua J, Skaltsounis A-L, *et al.* Natural alkaloids intervening the insulin pathway: new hopes for anti-diabetic agents? Curr Med Chem 2018; 25.
[http://dx.doi.org/10.2174/0929867325666180430152618]

[17]   Testa R, Bonfigli AR, Genovese S, *et al.* The possible role of flavonoids in the prevention of diabetic complications. Nutrients 2016; 8.
[http://dx.doi.org/10.3390/nu8050310]

[18]   Cherian S, Kumar RV, Augusti KT, Kidwai JR. Antidiabetic effect of a glycoside of pelargonidin isolated from the bark of Ficus bengalensis Linn. Indian J Biochem Biophys 1992; 29(4): 380-2.
[PMID: 1427968]

[19]   Patel DK, Prasad SK, Kumar R, Hemalatha S. An overview on antidiabetic medicinal plants having insulin mimetic property. Asian Pac J Trop Biomed 2012; 2(4): 320-30.
[http://dx.doi.org/10.1016/S2221-1691(12)60032-X] [PMID: 23569923]

[20]   Mellitus D, Jena PK. Nutritional and pharmacological importances of genus costus: a review. Int J Pharm Sci Res 2016; 7: 1866-73.

[21]   Behera A, Kumar S, Jena PK. Nutritional and pharmacological importances of genus costus: A review. Int J Pharm Sci Res 2016; 7: 1866-73.

[22]   Tchamgoue AD, Tchokouaha LRY, Tarkang PA, Kuiate JR, Agbor GA. *Costus afer* possesses carbohydrate hydrolyzing enzymes inhibitory activity and antioxidant capacity *in vitro*. Evid Based Complement Alternat Med 2015; 2015987984
[http://dx.doi.org/10.1155/2015/987984] [PMID: 26246844]

[23]   Hegde PK, Rao HA, Rao PN. A review on Insulin plant (*Costus igneus* Nak). Pharmacogn Rev 2014; 8(15): 67-72.
[http://dx.doi.org/10.4103/0973-7847.125536] [PMID: 24600198]

[24]   Owolabi OJ, Omogbai EKI, Falodun A. Oxytocic effects of the aqueous leaf extract of *Costus lucanusianus* - family Costaceae on isolated non-pregnant rat uterus. Pak J Pharm Sci 2010; 23(2): 207-11.
[PMID: 20363701]

[25]   Ajithabai MD, Sreedevi S, Jayakumar G, Nair MS, Deepa PN, Rani SS. Phytochemical analysis radical scavenging activity of the extracts of *Costus picatus* Linn *Coccinia indica* W& A, two Ethnic Medicinal Plants used in the Treatment of Diabetes mellitus. Free Radicals and Antioxidants. 2011 1;1(1):77-83.

[26]   Mašković JM. Isolation and Identification of Nicotiflorin Leaves of *Costus spectabilis* (Fenzl) K. Schum. www.pelagiaresearchlibrary.com

[27]   Britto RM, Santos AL, Cruz JS, *et al.* Aqueous fraction from *Costus spiralis* (Jacq.) Roscoe leaf reduces contractility by impairing the calcium inward current in the mammalian myocardium. J Ethnopharmacol 2011; 138(2): 382-9.
[http://dx.doi.org/10.1016/j.jep.2011.09.013] [PMID: 21963557]

[28]   Bello OA, Ayanda OI, Aworunse OS, *et al. Solanecio biafrae*: an underutilized nutraceutically-important african indigenous vegetable. Pharmacogn Rev 2018; 1: 1-9.

[29]   Simpson MG. Plant Systematics.Plant Systematics. Academic Press 2010; pp. 3-16.
[http://dx.doi.org/10.1016/B978-0-12-374380-0.50001-4]

[30]   Ajayakumar A, Sini KR, Sreekanth MC. Chemical and medico biological applications of the genus Costus (Gingers). J Chem Pharm Res 2016; 8: 453-8.

[31]   George A, Thankamma A, Rema Devi VK, *et al.* Phytochemical investigation of insulin plant (*Costus pictus*). Asian J Chem 2007; 19: 3427-30.

[32]   Devendran G, Sivamani G. Phytochemical Analysis Of Leaf Extract Of Plant Costus Spicatus By Gcms Method. J Drug Deliv Ther 2015; 5.
[http://dx.doi.org/10.22270/jddt.v5i4.1160]

[33]   Anyasor G, Obukohwo E, Adenike O. Bioactive compounds in *Costus afer* Ker Gawl leaves and stem fractions protect against calcium ion-induced mitochondrial membrane permeability transition. Oxid Antioxid Med Sci 2017; 6: 63.
[http://dx.doi.org/10.5455/oams.070917.or.111]

[34]   El-Far AH, Shaheen HM, Alsenosy AW, *et al. Costus speciosus*: Traditional uses, phytochemistry, and therapeutic potentials. Pharmacogn Rev 2018; 12: 120-7.
[http://dx.doi.org/10.4103/phrev.phrev_29_17]

[35]   Jayasri MA, Gunasekaran S, Radha A, *et al.* Anti-diabetic effect of *Costus pictus* leaves in normal and streptozotocin-induced diabetic rats. Int J Diabetes Metab 2008; 16: 117-22.

[36]   Jothivel N, Ponnusamy SP, Appachi M, *et al.* Anti-diabetic activity of methanol leaf extract of *Costus pictus* D. DON in alloxan-induced diabetic rats. J Health Sci 2007; 53: 655-63.
[http://dx.doi.org/10.1248/jhs.53.655]

[37]   Gireesh G, Thomas SK, Joseph B, Paulose CS. Antihyperglycemic and insulin secretory activity of *Costus pictus* leaf extract in streptozotocin induced diabetic rats and in *in vitro* pancreatic islet culture. J Ethnopharmacol 2009; 123(3): 470-4.
[http://dx.doi.org/10.1016/j.jep.2009.03.026] [PMID: 19501280]

[38]   Jayasri MA, Mathew L, Radha A. A report on the antioxidant activity of leaves and rhizomes of *Costus pictus* D. Don Plant material. Int J Integr Biol 2009; 5: 20-6.

[39]   Jayasri MA, Radha A, Mathew TL. A -Amylase and A -Glucosidase Inhibitory Activity of *Costus pictus* D. Don in the Management of Diabetes 2009; 3: 91-4.

[40]   Al-Romaiyan A, Jayasri MA, Mathew TL, *et al. Costus pictus* extracts stimulate insulin secretion from mouse and human islets of Langerhans *in vitro*. Cell Physiol Biochem 2010; 26(6): 1051-8.
[http://dx.doi.org/10.1159/000324007] [PMID: 21220936]

[41]   Ezejiofor AN, Orish CN, Orisakwe OE. Morphological changes in the pancreas and glucose reduction of the aqueous extract of *Costus afer* leaf on alloxan-induced diabetic rats. J Basic Clin Physiol Pharmacol 2015; 26(6): 595-601.
[http://dx.doi.org/10.1515/jbcpp-2014-0033] [PMID: 25514330]

[42]   Tchamgoue AD, Tchokouaha LRY, Tsabang N, Tarkang PA, Kuiate JR, Agbor GA. *Costus afer* Protects Cardio-, Hepato-, and Reno-Antioxidant Status in Streptozotocin-Intoxicated Wistar Rats. BioMed Res Int 2018; 20184907648
[http://dx.doi.org/10.1155/2018/4907648] [PMID: 30596093]

[43]   Tchamgoue AD, Tchokouaha LRY, Domekouo UL, *et al.* Effect of *Costus afer* on Carbohydrates Tolerance Tests and Glucose Uptake. Sch Acad J Biosci 2016; 4: 459-69.
[http://dx.doi.org/10.21276/sajb.2016.4.6.2]

[44]   Barminas JT, Onyema AM, Onwuka JC, *et al.* The Physicochemical, Toxicity and Anti-Diabetic Effect of *Costus afer* Ker Gawl. (Costaceae) Leaf Methanol Extract and Snail Slime on Alloxan Induced White Swiss Albino Rat. AASCIT J Chem 2017; 3: 23-9.

[45]   Uwah AF, Ewere EG, Ndem JI. Hypoglycemic and haematologic effects of crude stem juice of *Costus afer* on alloxaninduced diabetic wistar rats. American Journal of Ethnomedicine. 2015;2(4):2348-9502.

[46]   Monago C, Anacletus FC, Nwauche TK. Hypoglycaemic Activity of the aqueous extract of *Costus afer* stems alone and in combination with metformin. FASEB J 2016; 30: 1101-3.

[47]   Ezejiofor AN, Igweze ZN, Udowelle NA, Orisakwe OE. Histopathological and biochemical assessments of *Costus afer* stem on alloxan-induced diabetic rats. J Basic Clin Physiol Pharmacol 2017; 28(4): 383-91.
[http://dx.doi.org/10.1515/jbcpp-2016-0039] [PMID: 28355145]

[48]   Eliza J, Daisy P, Ignacimuthu S, Duraipandiyan V. Antidiabetic and antilipidemic effect of eremanthin from *Costus speciosus* (Koen.)Sm., in STZ-induced diabetic rats. Chem Biol Interact 2009; 182(1): 67-72.
[http://dx.doi.org/10.1016/j.cbi.2009.08.012] [PMID: 19695236]

[49]   Eliza J, Daisy P, Ignacimuthu S. Antioxidant activity of costunolide and eremanthin isolated from *Costus speciosus* (Koen ex. Retz) Sm. Chem Biol Interact 2010; 188(3): 467-72.
[http://dx.doi.org/10.1016/j.cbi.2010.08.002] [PMID: 20709041]

[50]   Rajesh MS, Harish MS, Sathyaprakash RJ, *et al.* Antihyperglycemic activity of the various extracts of *Costus speciosus* rhizomes. J Nat Rem 2009; 9: 235-41.

[51]   An experimental evaluation of the antidiabetic and antioxidant effect of *Costus speciosus* rhizome extract in alloxan induced albino rats. Biosci Biotechnol Res Asia 2011; 8: 789-93.
[http://dx.doi.org/10.13005/bbra/936]

[52]   Ali HA, Almaghrabi OA, Afifi ME. Molecular mechanisms of anti-hyperglycemic effects of *Costus speciosus* extract in streptozotocin-induced diabetic rats. Saudi Med J 2014; 35(12): 1501-6.
[PMID: 25491216]

[53]   Amila Sewwandi SHW, Menik HL, Sampath G, *et al.* Methanol and water extracts of *Costus speciosus* (j.kã–nig) sm. Leaves reverse the high fat diet induced peripheral insulin resistance in experimental wistar rats. Int Res J Pharm 2014; 5: 44-9.
[http://dx.doi.org/10.7897/2230-8407.050209]

[54]   Widiastuti EL. Ameliorative properties of crude diosgenin from *Costus speciosus* and taurine on testicular disorders in alloxan-induced diabetic mice. Biomed Pharmacol J 2017; 10: 9-17.
[http://dx.doi.org/10.13005/bpj/1075]

[55]   Alamoudi EF, Khalil WKB, Ghaly IS, *et al.* Nanoparticles from of *Costus speciosus* extract improves the antidiabetic and antilipidemic effects against STZ-induced diabetes mellitus in albino rats. Int J Pharm Sci Rev Res 2014; 29: 279-88.

[56]   Peasari J reddy, Motamarry S sri, Varma KS, et al. Chromatographic analysis of phytochemicals in *Costus igneus* and computational studies of flavonoids. Informatics Med Unlocked 2018; 13: 34-40.

[57]   Shetty AJ, Choudhury D, Rejeesh , Nair V, Kuruvilla M, Kotian S. Effect of the insulin plant (*Costus igneus*) leaves on dexamethasone-induced hyperglycemia. Int J Ayurveda Res 2010; 1(2): 100-2.
[http://dx.doi.org/10.4103/0974-7788.64396] [PMID: 20814523]

[58]   Reads C. Antidiabetic activity of insulin plant (*Costus igneus*) leaf extract in diabetic rats. 2016; 2-6.

[59]   Talasila E, Bavirisetti H, Chimakurthy J, *et al.* Effect of *Costus igneus*: The insulin plant, on prediabetes and diabetes in neonatal streptozotocin rats. J Health Sci 2014; 4: 162-8.
[http://dx.doi.org/10.17532/jhsci.2014.163]

[60]   Kanivalan N, Rajakumar R, Mani P. Anti-Diabetic and hypolipidamic effects of *Costus igneus* leaves extracts against streptozotocin induced diabetic albino rats. Acta Biomed Sci 2014; 1: 74-9.

[61]   Duarte RC, Taleb-Contini SH, Pereira PS, *et al.* Effect of *Costus spiralis* (Jacq.) Roscoe Leaves, Methanolic Extract and Guaijaverin on Blood Glucose and Lipid Levels in a Type II Diabetic Rat Model. Chem Biodivers 2019; 16(1)e1800365
[http://dx.doi.org/10.1002/cbdv.201800365] [PMID: 30371987]

[62]   de Oliveira AP, Coppede JS, Bertoni BW, *et al. Costus spiralis* (Jacq.) roscoe: a novel source of flavones with α-Glycosidase inhibitory activity. Chem Biodivers 2018; 15(1)e1700421
[http://dx.doi.org/10.1002/cbdv.201700421] [PMID: 29124880]

[63]   Kalailingam P, Devi Sekar A, Clement Samuel JS, *et al.* The efficacy of *Costus igneus* rhizome on carbohydrate metabolic, hepatoproductive and antioxidative enzymes in streptozotocin-induced diabetic rats. J Health Sci 2011; 57: 37-46.
[http://dx.doi.org/10.1248/jhs.57.37]

CHAPTER 5

Antidiabetic and Antihypertensive Potential of *Passiflora* spp. (Passion Fruit) - An Updated Review

Bency Baby T.[*] and **T.N.K. Suriyaprakash**

Department of Pharmacognosy, Al Shifa College of Pharmacy, Perintalmanna, Kerala - 679325, India

Abstract: Herbal medicines have been in use since stone days as an alternative therapy for the treatment of number of diseases. In this chapter, medicinal application of *Passiflora* genus in the treatment of diabetes mellitus, hypertension and related anxiety disorders are discussed. *Passiflora* belongs to the genera of Passifloraceae family. Species of the *Passiflora* fruits are edible and other parts of the plant including leaves, seeds, flowers and fruit peel are used in traditional system of medicine. Phyto constituents namely, Flavonoids, glycosides, phenolic compounds, alkaloids and volatile constituents are reported. Various studies carried out in the recent years reported various biological activities in the genus, including antioxidant, diuretic, anxiolytic, anti-inflammatory, analgesic, and antiviral properties. They also exhibited hypoglycemic, antihypertensive and antianxiety properties. The focus of this review is to preset the current state of knowledge and research findings associated with the use of the *Passiflora* species in the treatment of hyperglycemia and hypertension. Co-presence of diabetes mellitus and hypertension increases the risk of many health problems. In this chapter, we reviewed the findings of various species *viz. Passiflora edulis, Passiflora alata, Passiflora ligularis, Passiflora quadrangularis, Passiflora glandulosa, Passiflora incarnata*, Passiflora nitida, Passiflora nepalensis with the above mentioned activities. This chapter also aims to provide latest information on the medicinal benefits of *Passiflora* species which can be helpful to prevent hyperglycemia and related manifestation of Type 2 diabetes and hypertension.

Keywords: Antidiabetic potential, α amylse, α Glucosidase, Hypertension, *Passiflora*, Type 2 Diabetes.

INTRODUCTION

Diabetes and hypertension are both considered as major public health challenges

---

[*] **Corresponding author Bency Baby T:** Department of Pharmacognosy, Al Shifa College of Pharmacy, Poonthanam Post, Kizhattur, Perinthalmanna, Kerala – 679325, India; E-mail: bencybabyt@gmail.com

globally. Diabetes mellitus (DM) is a metabolic disorder in which abnormal level of blood sugar levels occur as a result of partial or complete lack of insulin secretion [1 - 3]. This may also result in other complications such as retinopathy, neuropathy, and nephropathy. DM is generally classified as type I and type II diabetes. Type I diabetes is (autoimmune disease or due to mutation), results from absolute deficiency in the production of insulin due to destroying beta (β) cells of pancreases. Type I represents only 10% of all diabetic cases, it affects all age groups, but the majority is more than 5 years. Type II diabetes is also known as non-insulin dependent diabetes mellitus. Type II is a common form of DM, which accounts for more than 80%, results from insulin deficiency or insulin resistance. Other minor types of DM are gestational diabetes mellitus (GDM), occur during pregnancy due to high blood glucose concentration. Currently, although type I cannot be prevented, type II is preventable with good health, exercising and healthy diet. Type II affected high population and led to complications in several body parts, heart, nerves, eyes, kidney and so on. Diabetes or hyperglycemia increases vulnerability to mortality and morbidity in patients. Diabetes may induce several other health related microvascular and macrovascular complications or could exist with other diseases. The macrovascular leads to more severe diseases like coronary disease, stroke and peripheral neuropathy. The microvascular are more erratic and in long-term may lead on macrovascular complications are diabetic retinopathy, diabetic nephropathy and diabetic foot. The clinical management of diabetic patients, health professionals combat with diabetic complications which are very common and come in broad spectrum of manifestations. The prevalence of diabetes has increased in adults and it raises the global public health burden and in another decade it can be predicted that India, China and USA will have the largest number of people affected with type II diabetes [4 - 7].

According to the World Health Organization, the clinical presentation of hypertension, which scientifically indicates the increase of blood pressure, has been defined as systolic (SBP)/diastolic (DBP) blood pressures of $\geq 140/90$ mmHg [8]. There are basically two types of hypertension. Primary hypertension, which accounts for about 95% of cases, usually has no traceable cause. Secondary hypertension associated with endocrine diseases, kidney disease, glucose intolerance and obesity. As it is commonly known that hypertension is related with several cardiovascular diseases such as arteriosclerosis, coronary artery disease, and myocardium infarction, renal insufficiency, stroke and dissecting aneurysm of aorta and if, hypertension, not promptly managed, results in decreasing ventricular function and, consequently, in heart failure. It is related to changed lifestyle and dietary habits that led to advanced cardiovascular events and arteriosclerosis both of which are linked with high blood pressure. Gender, age, socio-demographic characteristics and geographical location could also promote hypertension prevalence. Among the comprehensive lifestyle modifications, better dietary habits are one of the most effective measures for keeping hypertension under control [8 - 11].

The correlation among insulin resistance, diabetes and hypertension are complex and interrelated. It is estimated that about 25–47% of persons with hypertension have insulin resistance or impaired glucose tolerance. Correlation may be due to a common genetic and environmental factor promoting both diabetes and hypertension which along with obesity have been documented in several populations. Resistance to Insulin, renin-angiotensin-aldosterone system, endothelial dysfunction, and autonomic nervous system dysfunction play an important part in the pathogenesis of hypertension and diabetes [3].

Biguanides, Sulphonylureas, Glinides, Thiazolidinediones serves as oral hypoglycemic agents which are available along with insulin for the treatment of diabetes [4], while for hypertension, ACE inhibitors, Ang II receptor blockers, beta blockers, calcium channel blockers, renin inhibitors and diuretics are the common drugs. But side effects associated with their uses are reported. ACE inhibitors and diuretics are usually the first line of drugs in hypertension, which reduces the risk of kidney failure and cardiovascular events. However at the same time, these anti-hypertensive drugs are used in combination with anti-diabetic drugs, which may cause drug interactions and increase the risk of drugs-associated side effects in patients with diabetic and hypertension [12 - 14].

Similarly patients with anxiety disorders had a higher prevalence and a higher incidence of hypertension than that in the general population. Age, male sex, diabetes, and hyperlipidemia were risk factors for hypertension in patients with anxiety disorders. The impact of stress on the individuals's health covers changes in blood pressure, heart rate and an increased risk of cardiovascular diseases such as coronary heart disease. The link between major depression, insomnia and anxiety disorders impairs the function of immune and cardiovascular systems. Selective serotonin (5-HT) reuptake inhibitors (SSRIs), including citalopram, sertraline, fluoxetine are currently first-line drug treatment options for most anxiety disorders as they are proposed to have a better benefit/risk ratio than any other form of current pharmacotherapy. Long-term use of these drugs causes multiple inevitable side effects or tolerance. Also there has been considerable popular interest in using natural extracts and plant preparations to treat anxiety. Moreover, herbal medicines are considered as alternative of synthetic drugs. Relevant literature were collected by searching the major scientific databases including PubMed, Sciencedirect, Medline and Google scholar for plant species of *Passiflora* that have been investigated for anti-diabetic and antihypertensive activity [15, 16].

PHYTOTHERAPY IN MANAGEMENT OF DIABETES AND HYPERTENSION

Phytotherapy has a growing interest in the management of hypertension and diabetes because of the effectiveness, minimal side effects in clinical experience and relatively low costs. The use of plant based products has long been a source of medicinal preparations and there have been many reports for using herbal medicines for the treatment of diabetes over the years. Furthermore, the number of scientific publications on the use of herbal medicine and for type 2 diabetes is continuously on the raise. Among the possible mechanisms of action of natural products in diabetes, such as the inhibition of á-glucosidase and α-amylase, the effects on glucose uptake and glucose transporters, the enhancement of insulin secretion and of pancreatic cell proliferation, the antioxidant activity and inhibition of protein tyrosine phosphatase activity [17, 18].

Scientists and alternate medicine experts recommended that the consumption of grains, fruits, and vegetables should be increased to prevent or treat diabetes and related diseases. Among the possible components are protein, fibers, and some compounds called antinutrients, such as phytic acid, tannins, lecithins, and inhibitors of enzymes and saponins. Carbohydrates-hydrolysing enzymes inhibitors plays an important role to reduce the intake of sugar by the reduction of their intestinal absorption [18 - 21].

The main objective of any hypertensive diabetic should be to initiate lifestyle changes including stress management. These changes should include nourishment of diet, weight management, regular physical activity, and cessation of smoking. Dietary approach should consist of low sodium, high potassium, low calorie (800–1,500 kcal/day) and high fiber diet, shown to be effective in lowering BP. Coupled with diet, increased physical exercises such as walking for 30–45 minutes three to five days a week, has been shown to improve lipid profiles, BP and insulin resistance [3].

The World Health Organization (WHO) recommended that traditional medicinal practice should be followed, especially in countries where access to conventional treatment of diabetes exists. The discovery of the widely used hypoglycemic drug, metformin (N,*N* Dimethyl Guanyl Guanidine) came from the traditional approach through the use of *Galega officinalis* [3, 22, 23]. One of the most common approaches to reduce the intake of sugar is by the reduction of their intestinal metabolism using carbohydrates hydrolysing enzymes inhibitors. Studies were carried out for the potential role of natural products namely α – amylase, α - glucosidase inhibitors and antioxidant products [18, 21]. Fiber-rich diets are associated with a reduced risk of diabetes and cardiovascular disease (CVD) and it is inversely related to insulin resistance (IR) [24 - 33]. Some studies reported that the consumption of fiber rich diets may reduce the risk of disease in people, especially the prevention of cardiovascular disease like hypertension, gastrointestinal diseases like colon cancer; hyperlipidemia, diabetes, and obesity among others. Recently, many ayurvedic herbal formulations and other traditional medicinal systems are used in the treatment of diabetes mellitus and many ayurvedic products are being evaluated for their effectiveness in controlling diabetes [3, 19]. Many products from phytochemical sources have been identified or isolated against anti-diabetic and anti-hypertensive disorders, which will act synergistically against these diseases. Phenolic acids (p-coumaric acid, chlorogenic acid) and flavonoids (quercetin, rutin and naringenin) were the most identified compounds. verbascoside, leucosceptoside A and isoacteoside isolated from *Clerodendrum bungei* reported as the potent dual-acting therapeutic compound. Therefore, it is essential to explore other avenues, such as ethnomedicine, for possible therapeutic agents, which may be helpful in the concomitant management of diabetes and hypertension, with less side effects [29].

THE GENUS *PASSIFLORA*

Kingdom: Plantae

Subkingdom: Tracheobionta

Superdivision: Spermatophyta

Division: Magnoliophyta

Class: Magnoliopsıda

Subclass: Dilleniidae

Order: Violales

Family: Passifloraceae

Genus: Passiflora

The genus *Passiflora* is the highest and most diverse of the family Passifloraceae, comprising more than 600 species of vines, lianas, trees and shrubs, commonly used for their fruits, ornamental and medicinal properties. The passion fruit (Fig. **1**) is the popular name given to several species of the genus *Passiflora*. The plants of this genus are mainly distributed in the hot and tropical temperate regions of the New World; they are much rarer in Asia, Australia and tropical

Africa. Several species are cultivated in the tropics for their edible fruits (Passion fruit or Purple Passion fruit). Many others are grown outdoors in the warmest parts of the world or in greenhouses for their exotic flowers. Some common *Passiflora* species are *P. edulis* (Purple Passion fruit), *P. incarnata (*Maypop), *P. foetida (*Stinking passion flower), *P. alata* (Winged stem passion flower), *P. actinia*, *P. quadrangularis* (Giant granadilla), *P. caerulae* (Blue passion flower) and *P. lutea* (yellow passion flower) [34 - 42].

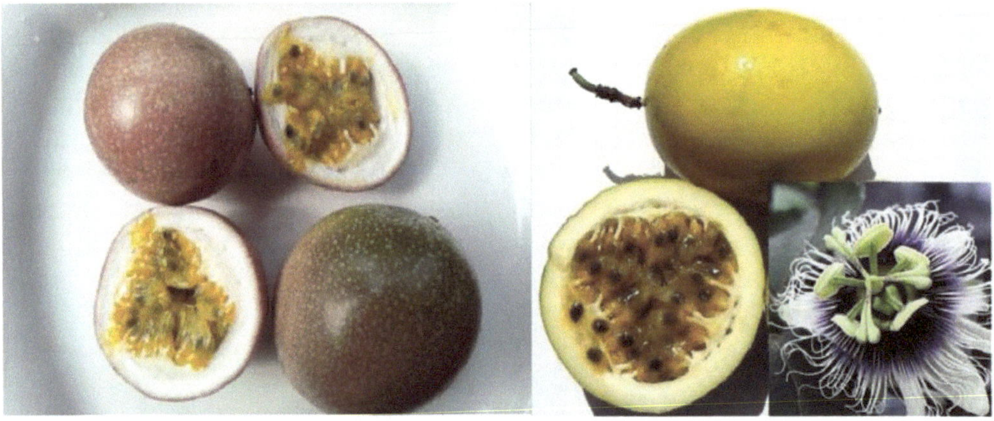

Fig. (1). Passion fruit and its flower.

Phytochemistry

The different parts of the plant, leaves, fruits and roots of the species of *Passiflora,* are traditionally used in several countries for the treatment of insomnia, anxiety and irritability. The domestic consumption of fruits, peels, teas and pulp of *Passiflora* are not uncommon. It is reported that the genus *Passiflora* contains alkaloids, flavonoids, phenolic compounds, cyanogenic compounds and polyamines. Polyphenolic compounds, especially flavonoids, are known as the most common chemical class of phytochemicals that possess a wide range of beneficial effects for health promotion [37, 43]. Flavonoids are the main phyto-constituents in many species and include apigenin (1), luteolin (2), quercetin (3), kaempferol [44]. Among the various Passiflora species of medicinal herbs *P. edulis* has been widely used in the traditional therapeutic system and has now become an official Pharmacopoeia component in several countries. It has been observed that many species contain betacarboline and harmala alkaloids [45 - 48]. The chemical structures of principle active constituents reported in Passiflora genus are given in Fig. (2). The leaf extract of the plant plays an important role in the neutralization of free radicals in the organism and, therefore, prevents diabetes mellitus. Some species of *Passiflora* have anxiolytic, sedative, antihypertensive, anti-inflammatory, cytotoxic, antibacterial and antifungal activity [37, 50]. Considering the importance of these species for treatment of diabetes mellitus and hypertension this chapter is a review of medicinal plants and natural products from genus *Passiflora*.

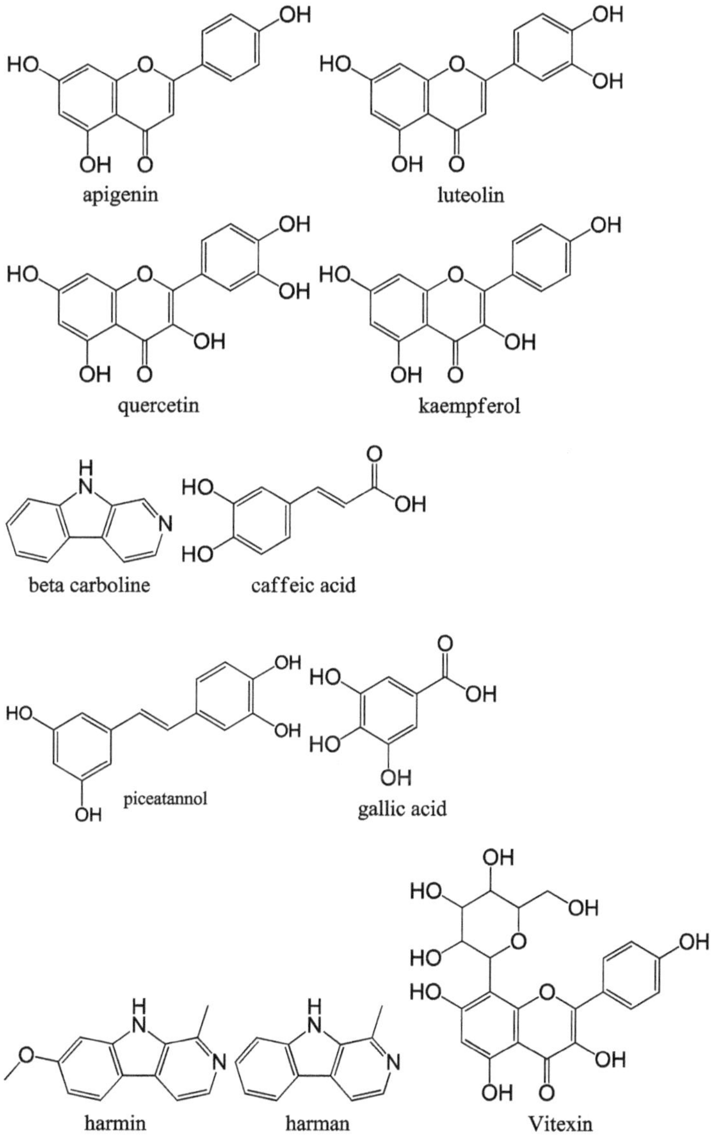

Fig. (2). Chemical structures of selected compounds isolated from *Passiflora* genus.

Antidiabetic Activity

Many *in vitro* and *in vivo* studies were undertaken by researchers to evaluate traditional and local anti-diabetic claims of passion fruit. The anti-diabetic properties of the passion fruit can be observed in the juice of the passion fruit, pectin, peel, flour, seeds and cellulose of the mesocarp. After treatment with passion fruit juice, wistar diabetic rats demonstrated the effect of preventing and treating dyslipidemia and hyperglycemia [51]. Colomeu *et al.* reported the potential benefits of aqueous leaf extract of *P. alata* (*P. alata*) in experimental type 1 diabetes. Different antioxidant responses obtained using DPPH; FRAP; ABTS; and ORAC analysis. The anti-inflammatory properties of extract were also studied. In experimental type 1 diabetes, non-obese diabetic mice were divided into two groups. The *P. alata* group was treated with aqueous extract of *P. alata* Curtis, and a non-treated control group, followed by diabetes expression analysis. The consumption of aqueous extract and water *ad libitum* lasted 7 months. The treated group presented reduced in diabetes incidence; a low quantity of infiltrative cells in pancreatic islets raised glutathione in the kidney and liver, when compared with the diabetic and non-diabetic control-groups. The study revealed that the aqueous extract has a higher antioxidant activity, due to its flavonoid compounds apigenin, vitexin, isovitexin and isoorientin. So, the intake of aqueous extract of *P. alata* may be considered a good source of natural antioxidants and compounds found in its composition can act as anti-inflammatory agents, helping in the control of diabetes by easing insulin resistance effect [52].

In type 2 diabetic patients, insulin resistance is the main cause of diabetics. Queiroz *et al.*, reported the antidiabetic effect of *Passiflora glandulosa (P. glandulosa)* fruit rinds flour on streptozotocin (STZ)-induced diabetic mice. A significant difference was observed in the fasting blood glucose after dietary supplemented yellow passion fruit peel flour [53]. Flavanones and triterpenoids are reported to be the major phytoconstituents of this flour which were responsible for the anti-diabetic activity, acting by increase of insulin release and by modifying the glucose metabolism in hepatocytes, as well as inhibiting the synthesis of enzymes in hepatocytes. It is also reported that the presence of fiber from *P. glandulosa* fruit rinds flour promoted satiety due to delayed gastric emptying; in this way, the reduction of carbohydrate intake may have improved insulin sensitivity and reduction of glycemia. Similarly, Passion fruit pectin was also reported to have hypoglycemic and hypotriglyceridemic properties in diabetic rats [53 - 56]. Morton reported that the basic nutrients such as protein, carbohydrates, amino acids, vitamins and fiber are present in *Passiflora ligularis* fruit pulp [6]. The fruit peel also possesses higher polysaccharides like xylose, glucose, galactose, galactosamine, and fructose [57]. Saravanan *et al.* reported anti-radical, anti-diabetic and activities of different solvent extracts of *P. ligularis* fruits. Different solvent extracts of fruit pulp was investigated using standard assays for antioxidant like DPPH, ABTS, hydroxyl, superoxide radical nitric oxide for testing the response. The acetone extract of *P. ligularis* fruits also exhibited significant (P<0.005) inhibition activities on α-amylase and α-glucosidase. α-glucosidase inhibition activity of fruit pulp may be due to its high phenolic, flavonoid contents and its antioxidant activity. Fruit pulp also contains gallic acid, caffeic acid, rutin, ellagic acid as the phenolic compounds [58]. Similarly in another study, in STZ-induced diabetic wistar rats, single oral dose (400 mg/kg body weight) of *P. ligularis* fruit extract showed a stronger blood glucose lowering effect [59]. Hypoglycemic activity *of P. ligularis* was quite comparable with reduction brought about by standard drug glibenclamide. In addition, the passion fruit seed showed anti-diabetic properties. An ingredient in the passion fruit seed, called piceatannol, can reduce fasting blood glucose levels [60].

Another study (Barbalho *et al.*) reported the positive results of *P. edulis fruit* juice on the biochemical profile of offspring from diabetic rats. After treatment diabetic wistar rat offspring showed the effect of preventing and treating dyslipidemia and hyperglycemia. The antidiabetic effect of passion fruit may be related to the compounds in its pulp like pectin, vitamin C, carotenoids, flavonoids and minerals. This plant may have beneficial effects in the prevention and treatment of dyslipidemia and hyperglycemia, it improves lipid profiles [51]. Gupta *et al.* (2012) studied and assessed the role of *Passiflora incarnata* leaf extracts for the treatment for diabetes. The methanolic extract exhibited significant hypoglycemic activity in STZ-diabetic mice, comparable to the effect exhibited by standard drug glibenclamide. The urine glucose level is used as the evidence for tolerance to oral glucose as well as the differences in serum lipid and body weight profiles, compared with diabetic mice treated with drugs. The histopathological studies of the animal pancreas showed considerable cell regeneration, induced by the *P. incarnata* extract after the cells were necrotic, due to the effect of the streptozotocin. In their investigation it was reported that activity of extract may be due to the stimulation of insulin release and increased peripheral glucose utilization. Flavanoid constitutes the active biological principle of most medicinal plants that have already been reported to have hypoglycemic activity. Methanol extract showed the presence of flavanoids, saponins, phenolic compounds and tannins making this plant a promising source for the future treatment of diabetes in humans. In patients with type 2 diabetes, insulin resistance is a major cause of diabetes, and it has been found that passion fruit flour reduces insulin resistance. A significant difference was observed in fasting blood glucose (P=0.000) and glycated hemoglobin (P=0.032) after adding yellow passion fruit flour to food [56, 61].

Pereira *et al.* described the antidiabetic effect of *Passiflora nitida* extract in an animal model of diabetes. The hydroethanolic leaf extract of the plant on *in vitro* α-glucosidase inhibitory activity showed an IC_{50} value of 6.78 μg/mL, whereas α-amylase inhibition, which is an important therapeutic target in the regulation of postprandial increase of blood glucose in diabetic patients the IC_{50} was found to be 93.36 μg/mL. The work also reports *in vivo* experiments in which the wistar rats were treated orally with 50 mg/kg of *P. nitida* extract and were compared to non-treated and non-diabetic rats. Results of different saccharide tolerance test manifested significant glycemia control and, with alloxan-diabetic mice, resulted in a decrease of total cholesterol, a hypoglycemic effect, and an antioxidant activity by thiobarbituric acid-reactive substances measurement. The results indicated its potential to inhibit enzymes involved in carbohydrate metabolism [62].

Antihypertensive Activity

In spite of advanced pharmacotherapy and mechanical treatments, cardiovascular disease remains a leading cause of morbidity and mortality worldwide. There are few experimental studies that have examined the effects of passion fruit on hypertension. *Passiflora edulis,* which is another species of *Passiflora,* has antihypertensive effects. It is used in folklore medicine for treating hypertension. Ichimura *et al.* reported that the oral administration of methanolic extract of purple passion fruit significantly reduces systolic and diastolic blood pressure in spontaneously hypertensive rats. Quantitative analysis by liquid chromatography tandem mass spectrometry (LC–MS/MS) demonstrated that extract contained luteolin-6-C-glucoside. It was also reported to contain gamma amino butyric acid (GABA, 2.4 mg/g dry weight by LC–MS/MS), which has been reported to be an antihypertensive material. The study proposed the antihypertensive effects of the extract in spontaneously hypertensive rats might be due the GABA-induced antihypertensive effect and partially to the vasodilatory effect of polyphenols including luteolin [63].

In another experimental study by Zibadi *et al.,* spontaneously hypertensive rats were fed diet supplemented with either 10 or 50 mg/kg purple passion fruit peel extract. The peel possesses high molecular weight polysaccharides like xylose, glucose, galactose, galactosamine, and fructose. It was an 8 weeks study where rats were split into three groups consisting of control and experimental. Researchers found that systolic blood pressure significantly lowered in rats fed the basic diet supplemented with 50 mg kg of passion fruit extract *versus* the controls. The effect of the treatment on immune parameters was also evaluated, which showed no statistical changes. Studies were then extended to hypertensive human subjects who were administered the passion fruit peel extract (400 mg/d) or placebo pills within a 4-weeks randomized, placebo-controlled, double-blind trial. The effects of the passion fruit peel extract were evaluated by blood pressure measurement. The systolic and diastolic blood pressure of the passion fruit peel extract–treated group decreased significantly by, compared with the placebo group. No adverse effect was reported by the patients. HPLC analysis identified the following major constituents cyanidin 3-*O*-glucoside, quercetin 3-O-glucoside, and edulilic acid, a novel cyclic acid glucoside from the extract. The results suggest that the antihypertensive effect of the passion fruit peel extract may, in part, be mediated through nitric oxide modulation. It is suggested that the PFP extract may be offered as a safe alternative treatment to hypertensive patients [64, 65].

Another study evaluated the antihypertensive effect of yellow passion fruit pulp which was administered to spontaneously hypertensive rats (SHR). The safety of yellow passion fruit pulp consumption was studied and also mechanisms responsible for its antihypertensive action were discussed. The effect of this pulp has been evaluated for kidney function because the kidneys are most affected by hypertension and are predominant in blood pressure homeostasis. HLPC-PDA-MS/MS analysis revealed that yellow passion fruit pulp contains phenolic compounds, ascorbic acid, carotenoids and flavonoids. The study reported that the antihypertensive effect of yellow passion fruit pulp might be due to the enhancement of the antioxidant status [66].

Another *in vivo* study disclosed the effects of passion fruit juice. In this work hypertensive patient intervened with *P. edulis* juice. This study revealed the effect of *P. edulis* juice on blood pressure, angiotensin converting enzyme activity, oxidative stress and blood lipids in non-chronic hypertensive patients. This intervention reduced systolic and diastolic pressure (142.4 to 125.2 mm Hg and 79 to 76.1 mmHg, respectively. compared to the group not intervened (139.5 to 134.9 and 89.7 to 84.0 mmHg, respectively. Although *P. edulis* juice consumption does not protect against hemolysis, it increases the antioxidant capacity of patients' serum. Polyphenols, especially flavonoids, have shown antihypertensive effect in different experimental models thus, for example, in *in-vivo* models, using hypertensive rats, the flavonoid quercetin induced a significant reduction in systolic, diastolic, and mean blood pressure [67].

Passiflora incarnata L. is important in herbal medicine for treating anxiety related problems, hypertension, sexual dysfunction and menopause. Another study communicated the *in vitro* effects of a dry extract of *P.incarnata* on the GABA system. The extract inhibited [3H]-GABA uptake into rat cortical synaptosomes but had no effect on GABA release and GABA transaminase activity. *P.incarnata* inhibited concentration dependently the binding of [3H]- SR95531 to GABAA-receptors and of [3H]-CGP 54626 to GABAB-receptors. Using the [35S]-GTPgS binding assay *Passiflora* could be classified as an antagonist of the GABAB receptor. In contrast, the ethanol- and the benzodiazepine-site of the GABAA-receptor were not affected by this extract. The researchers concluded that numerous pharmacological effects of *P. incarnata* are mediated *via* modulation of the GABA system including affinity to GABAA and GABAB receptors, and effects on GABA uptake [68].

Passiflora nepalensis is another plant used in folklore medicine for treating hypertension . Chemical constituents of this plant include phenolic compounds, alkaloids, glycosyl flavonoids which possess antioxidant activity. A study has been conducted by Patel *et al.* in which they have demonstrated that the aqueous extract of the *P. nepelensis* posses strong antihypertensive activity. In another study researchers have found that the methanolic extract of the whole plant of *P. nepalensis* plant lowered the blood pressure and heart rate of hypertensive rats which clearly shows that this plant possesses strong antihypertensive property [69].

Bareno *et al.* communicated the effect of *Passiflora quadrangularis* L. ethanolic extract in experimental hypertension induced in wistar rats. *P. quadrangularis* prevented experimental hypertension induced in rats with nitric oxide deficits improving the endothelium vasodilatation response and protecting against vascular remodelling. Phytochemical studies of *Passiflora* species have led to isolation of the indole alkaloids: such as harmalol, harmol, harmane, harmaline and harmine, and the C glycosyl flavonoids: orientin, isoorientin, vitexin, and isovitexin. In addition flavonoids, triterpene glycoside saponins, some cycloartenol type, have also been identified from the species mentioned in this chapter. However more studies are required in this direction [70].

CONCLUSION

The present chapter reports the main and important pharmacological activities of *Passiflora* genus in controlling diabetes and hypertension. Recent research has provided a scientific basis for traditional medicine, and confirmed its importance in the prevention and treatment of diabetes and hypertension and their associated disorders. The extensive literature survey, based on the knowledge and experience of preclinical, clinical and human studies has revealed its potential and it is logical to assume that, among the Passifloracea members many of them are having anti-hypertensive and antidiabetic activity. Phenolic acids (gallic acid, ellagic acid, caffeic acid) and flavonoids (quercetin, rutin, apigenin, vitexin, isovitexin, kaempferol) are the important phytoconstituents present in the plants under review. Alkaloids (harmine, harman, harmaline, harmine), piceatannol, betacarboline, pectin were also reported from the species mentioned in this chapter. However, the precise underlying mechanisms of action still remained to be determined. It is recommended that such antidiabetic and anti-hypertensive investigations of medicinal plants, with effect comparable to standard drugs, be completely conducted from *in vitro* to *in vivo* experimental conditions, with concomitant toxicity studies to ascertain the safety profile. The dual antidiabetic and antihypertensive action of medicinal plants present a fascinating opportunity for the development of therapeutic bioactive preparations or pure bioactive compounds for the simultaneous management of diabetes and hypertension. In this chapter, the relevant literature concludes that medicinal plants could also serve as a potential source to develop dual action therapies against diabetes and hypertension but more extensive research needs to be done.

CONSENT FOR PUBLICATION

Not applicable.

CONFLICT OF INTEREST

There is no conflict of interest declared.

ACKNOWLEDGEMENT

Declared none.

REFERENCES

[1]   Klein O, Lynge J, Endahl L, Damholt B, Nosek L, Heise T. Albumin-bound basal insulin analogues (insulin detemir and NN344): comparable time-action profiles but less variability than insulin glargine in type 2 diabetes. Diabetes Obes Metab 2007; 9(3): 290-9.
        [http://dx.doi.org/10.1111/j.1463-1326.2006.00685.x] [PMID: 17391154]

[2]   Surya S, Salam AD, Tommy DV, Carla B, Kumar RA. Diabetes mellitus and medicinal plants-review. Asian Pac J Trop Dis 2014; 4(5): 337-47.
        [http://dx.doi.org/10.1016/S2222-1808(14)60585-5]

[3]   Shanmugam S, Rajan M, de Souza AA. Araújo, Narain N. Potential of Passion (*Passiflora Spp.*) Fruit in Control of Type II Diabetes. Curr Res Diabetes Obes J 2018; 7(3)555712

[4]   Tabeshpour J, Razavi BM, Hosseinzadeh H. Effects of Avocado (*Persea americana*) on Metabolic Syndrome: A Comprehensive Systematic Review. Phytother Res 2017; 31(6): 819-37.
        [http://dx.doi.org/10.1002/ptr.5805] [PMID: 28393409]

[5]   Smith CJ, Ryckman KK. Epigenetic and developmental influences on the risk of obesity, diabetes, and metabolic syndrome. Diabetes Metab Syndr Obes 2015; 8: 295-302.
        [http://dx.doi.org/10.2147/DMSO.S61296] [PMID: 26170704]

[6]   Wild S, Roglic G, Green A, Sicree R, King H. Global prevalence of diabetes: estimates for the year 2000 and projections for 2030. Diabetes Care 2004; 27(5): 1047-53.
        [http://dx.doi.org/10.2337/diacare.27.5.1047] [PMID: 15111519]

[7]   Okur ME, *et al.* Diabetes mellitus: A review on pathophysiology, current status of oral medications and future perspectives. Acta Pharm Sci 2017; 55: 61-82.

[8]   Abdul Rashid A, Khalid Y, Chia Y. Management of hypertension. Malays Fam Physician 2011; 6(1): 40-3.
[PMID: 25606222]

[9]   Hügel HM, Jackson N, May B, Zhang AL, Xue CC. Polyphenol protection and treatment of hypertension. Phytomedicine 2016; 23(2): 220-31.
[http://dx.doi.org/10.1016/j.phymed.2015.12.012] [PMID: 26926184]

[10]   Wengreen H, Munger RG, Cutler A, *et al.* Prospective study of dietary approaches to stop hypertension-and Mediterranean-style dietary pat-terns and age-related cognitive change: The Cache county study on memory, health and aging. Am J Clin Nutr 2013; 98(5): 1263-71.
[http://dx.doi.org/10.3945/ajcn.112.051276] [PMID: 24047922]

[11]   Okur ME, Karantas ID, Okur NU, Siafaka PI. Hypertension in 2017: update in treatment and pharmaceutical innovations. Curr Pharm Des 2017; 23(44): 6795-814.
[http://dx.doi.org/10.2174/1381612823666170927123454] [PMID: 28969533]

[12]   Holman RR, Turner RC. Oral Agents and insulin in the treatment of Diabetes, Blackwell publication, Oxford. 1991, 467-469.

[13]   Mamakou V, Eleftheriadou I, Katsiki N, Makrilakis K, Tsioufis K, Tentolouris N. Antidiabetic Drugs as Antihypertensives: New Data on the Horizon. Curr Vasc Pharmacol 2017; 16(1): 70-8.
[http://dx.doi.org/10.2174/1570161115666171010122332] [PMID: 29032756]

[14]   Whalen KL, Stewart RD. Pharmacologic management of hypertension in patients with diabetes. Am Fam Physician 2008; 78(11): 1277-82.
[PMID: 19069021]

[15]   Simone B. Novel pharmacological targets in drug development for the treatment of anxiety and anxiety-related disorders Pharmacology & Therapeutics 2019.: 107402..

[16]   Wu EL, Chien IC, Lin CH. Increased risk of hypertension in patients with anxiety disorders: a population-based study. J Psychosom Res 2014; 77(6): 522-7.
[http://dx.doi.org/10.1016/j.jpsychores.2014.10.006] [PMID: 25454679]

[17]   Governa P, Baini G, Borgonetti V, *et al.* Phytotherapy in the management of diabetes: a review. Molecules 2018; 23(1)E105
[http://dx.doi.org/10.3390/molecules23010105] [PMID: 29300317]

[18]   Loizzo MR, Lucci P, Núñez O, *et al.* Native colombian fruits and their by-products: Phenolic profile, antioxidant activity and hypoglycaemic potential. Foods 2019; 8(3): 89.
[http://dx.doi.org/10.3390/foods8030089] [PMID: 30832443]

[19]   Salgado JM, Bombarde TA, Mansi DN, Piedade SMS, Meletti LMM. Effects of different concentrations of passion fruit peel (*Passiflora edulis*) on the glicemic control in diabetic rat. Food Sci Technol (Campinas) 2010; 30(3): 784-9.
[http://dx.doi.org/10.1590/S0101-20612010000300034]

[20]   Diet and Health Implications for reducing chronic disease risk. Washington, D.C.: National Academy Press 1989.

[21]   Loizzo MR, Bonesi M, Nabavi SM, Sobarzo-Sánchez E, Rastrelli L, Tundis R. Hypoglycaemic effects of plants food constituents *via* inhibition of carbohydrate-hydrolysing enzymes: From chemistry to future applications. Nat Prod Target Clin Relev Enzym 2017; 1: 135-61.
[http://dx.doi.org/10.1002/9783527805921.ch6]

[22]   Almeida JRGDS, Souza GR, Araujo ECDC, *et al.* Medicinal plants and natural compounds from the genus *Morus* (Moraceae) with hypoglycemic activity: a review. In: Chackrewarthy S, Ed. Glucose Tolerance. Intech Open 2012; pp. 189-206.
[http://dx.doi.org/10.5772/53145]

[23]   Grover JK, Yadav S, Vats V. Medicinal plants of India with anti-diabetic potential. J Ethnopharmacol

2002; 81(1): 81-100.
[http://dx.doi.org/10.1016/S0378-8741(02)00059-4] [PMID: 12020931]

[24]   de Queiroz MdoS, Janebro DI, da Cunha MA, *et al.* Effect of the yellow passion fruit peel flour *(Passiflora edulis f. flavicarpa* deg.) in insulin sensitivity in type 2 diabetes mellitus patients. Nutr J 2012; 11(89): 89.
[http://dx.doi.org/10.1186/1475-2891-11-89] [PMID: 23088514]

[25]   Wannamethee SG, Whincup PH, Thomas MC, Sattar N. Associations between dietary fiber and inflammation, hepatic function, and risk of type 2 diabetes in older men: potential mechanisms for the benefits of fiber on diabetes risk. Diabetes Care 2009; 32(10): 1823-5.
[http://dx.doi.org/10.2337/dc09-0477] [PMID: 19628814]

[26]   Schulze MB, Schulz M, Heidemann C, Schienkiewitz A, Hoffmann K, Boeing H. Fiber and magnesium intake and incidence of type 2 diabetes: a prospective study and meta-analysis. Arch Intern Med 2007; 167(9): 956-65.
[http://dx.doi.org/10.1001/archinte.167.9.956] [PMID: 17502538]

[27]   Hodge AM, English DR, O'Dea K, Giles GG. Glycemic index and dietary fiber and the risk of type 2 diabetes. Diabetes Care 2004; 27(11): 2701-6.
[http://dx.doi.org/10.2337/diacare.27.11.2701] [PMID: 15505008]

[28]   Barclay AW, Flood VM, Rochtchina E, Mitchell P, Brand-Miller JC. Glycemic index, dietary fiber, and risk of type 2 diabetes in a cohort of older Australians. Diabetes Care 2007; 30(11): 2811-3.
[http://dx.doi.org/10.2337/dc07-0784] [PMID: 17712022]

[29]   Chukwuma CI, Matsabisa MG, Ibrahim MA, Erukainure OL, Chabalala MH, Islam MS. Medicinal plants with concomitant anti-diabetic and anti-hypertensive effects as potential sources of dual acting therapies against diabetes and hypertension: A review. J Ethnopharmacol 2019; 235: 329-60.
[http://dx.doi.org/10.1016/j.jep.2019.02.024] [PMID: 30769039]

[30]   Galisteo M, Duarte J, Zarzuelo A. Effects of dietary fibers on disturbances clustered in the metabolic syndrome. J Nutr Biochem 2008; 19(2): 71-84.
[http://dx.doi.org/10.1016/j.jnutbio.2007.02.009] [PMID: 17618108]

[31]   Venn BJ, Mann JI. Cereal grains, legumes and diabetes. Eur J Clin Nutr 2004; 58(11): 1443-61.
[http://dx.doi.org/10.1038/sj.ejcn.1601995] [PMID: 15162131]

[32]   Fung TT, Hu FB, Pereira MA, *et al.* Whole-grain intake and the risk of type 2 diabetes: a prospective study in men. Am J Clin Nutr 2002; 76(3): 535-40.
[http://dx.doi.org/10.1093/ajcn/76.3.535] [PMID: 12197996]

[33]   Liu S, Manson JE, Stampfer MJ, *et al.* Whole grain consumption and risk of ischemic stroke in women: A prospective study. JAMA 2000; 284(12): 1534-40.
[http://dx.doi.org/10.1001/jama.284.12.1534] [PMID: 11000647]

[34]   J Simão M, J S Barboza T, G Vianna M, *et al.* A comparative study of phytoconstituents and antibacterial activity of *in vitro* derived materials of four *Passiflora* species. An Acad Bras Cienc 2018; 90(3): 2805-13.
[http://dx.doi.org/10.1590/0001-3765201820170809] [PMID: 30043909]

[35]   Ulmer Torsten, MacDougal John M. Passiflora: passionflowers of the world. Portland, Cambridge: Timber Press 2004.

[36]   http://plants.usda.gov/java/classification

[37]   Dhawan K, Dhawan S, Sharma A. *Passiflora*: a review update. J Ethnopharmacol 2004; 94(1): 1-23.
[http://dx.doi.org/10.1016/j.jep.2004.02.023] [PMID: 15261959]

[38]   The Wealth of India. A Dictionary of Indian Raw Materials and Industrial Products CSIR 9-278.

[39]   Sacco JC. Passifloráceas. In: Reitz R, Ed. Flora ilustrada catarinense. Itajaı, Brazil: Herbario Barbosa Rodrigues 1980; pp. 1-132.

[40]   Spencer KC, Seigler DS. Cyanogenesis of *Passiflora edulis*. J Agric Food Chem 1983; 31(4): 794-6.
[http://dx.doi.org/10.1021/jf00118a028] [PMID: 6619429]

[41]   Wohlmuth H, Penman KG, Pearson T, Lehmann RP. Pharmacognosy and chemotypes of passionflower (*Passiflora incarnata* L.). Biol Pharm Bull 2010; 33(6): 1015-8.
[http://dx.doi.org/10.1248/bpb.33.1015] [PMID: 20522969]

[42]   McGuire CM. *P. incarnata* (Passifloraceae): a new fruit crop. Econ Bot 1999; 53: 161-76.
[http://dx.doi.org/10.1007/BF02866495]

[43]   Gadioli IL, da Cunha MSB, de Carvalho MVO, Costa AM, Pineli LLO. A systematic review on phenolic compounds in *Passiflora* plants: Exploring biodiversity for food, nutrition, and popular medicine. Crit Rev Food Sci Nutr 2018; 58(5): 785-807.
[http://dx.doi.org/10.1080/10408398.2016.1224805] [PMID: 27645583]

[44]   Teixeira N, Jean C S. Edible fruits from Brazilian biodiversity: A review on their sensorial characteristics versus bioactivity as tool to select research 119. 2019; 325-48.

[45]   Parfitt K. Martindale: The Complete Drug Reference. 32nd ed. London: Pharmaceutical Press 1999; p. 1570.

[46]   Ingale AG, Hivrale AU. Pharmacological studies of *Passiflora* sp. and their bioactive compounds. Afr J Plant Sci 2010; 41(10): 417-26.

[47]   Hiremath SP, Badami S, Hunasagatta SK, Patil SB. Antifertility and hormonal properties of flavones of *Striga orobanchioides*. Eur J Pharmacol 2000; 391(1-2): 193-7.
[http://dx.doi.org/10.1016/S0014-2999(99)00723-2] [PMID: 10720651]

[48]   Rehwald A, Meier BE, Sticher O. Qualitative and quantitative reversed phase high-performance liquid chromatography of flavonoids in *Passiflora incarnata* L. Pharm Acta Helv 1994; 69: 153-8.
[http://dx.doi.org/10.1016/0031-6865(94)90017-5]

[49]   Raffaelli A, Moneti G, Mercati V, Toja E. Mass spectrometric characterization of flavonoids in extracts from *Passiflora incarnata*. J Chromatogr A 1997; 777: 223-31.
[http://dx.doi.org/10.1016/S0021-9673(97)00260-4]

[50]   Ramaiya Shiamala Devi, Bujang Japar Sidik, Zakaria Muta Harah. Assessment oftotal phenolic, antioxidant, and antibacterial activities of Passiflora species. 2014.

[51]   Barbalho SM, Damasceno DC, Spada AP, *et al.* Effects of *Passiflora edulis* on the metabolic profile of diabetic Wistar rat offspring. J Med Food 2011; 14(12): 1490-5.
[http://dx.doi.org/10.1089/jmf.2010.0318] [PMID: 21663518]

[52]   Colomeu TC, Figueiredo D, Cazarin CB, *et al.* Antioxidant and anti-diabetic potential of *Passiflora alata* Curtis aqueous leaves extract in type 1 diabetes mellitus (NOD-mice). Int Immunopharmacol 2014; 18(1): 106-15.
[http://dx.doi.org/10.1016/j.intimp.2013.11.005] [PMID: 24269180]

[53]   Queiroz EM, Paim RT, Lira SM, *et al.* Antihyperglycemic effect of *Passiflora glandulosa* cav. fruit rinds flour in streptozotocin-induced diabetic mice. Asian Pac J Trop Med 2018; 11: 510.
[http://dx.doi.org/10.4103/1995-7645.242308]

[54]   Silva RO, Damasceno SR, Brito TV, *et al.* Polysaccharide fraction isolated from *Passiflora edulis* inhibits the inflammatory response and the oxidative stress in mice. J Pharm Pharmacol 2015; 67(7): 1017-27.
[http://dx.doi.org/10.1111/jphp.12399] [PMID: 25808583]

[55]   Dornas WC, De Oliveira TT, Dores RGR, Fabres MHA, Nagem TJ. Efeitos antidiabeticos de plantas medicinais. Braz J Pharmacog 2009; 19(2A): 488-500.
[http://dx.doi.org/10.1590/S0102-695X2009000300024]

[56]   Pereira MA, Ludwig DS. Dietary fiber and body-weight regulation. Observations and mechanisms. Pediatr Clin North Am 2001; 48(4): 969-80.

[http://dx.doi.org/10.1016/S0031-3955(05)70351-5] [PMID: 11494646]

[57]   Morton JF. Passifloraceae Fruits of Warm Climates; Miami, FL: JF 1987; 320-8.

[58]   Saravanan S, Parimelazhagan T. *In vitro* antioxidant, antimicrobial and anti-diabetic properties of polyphenols of *Passiflora ligularis* Juss. fruit pulp. Food Sci Hum Wellness 2014; 3: 56-64.
[http://dx.doi.org/10.1016/j.fshw.2014.05.001]

[59]   Anusooriya P, Malarvizhi D, Gopalakrishnan V K, Devaki K. Antioxidant andantidiabetic effect of aqueous fruit extract of *Passiflora ligularis* Juss. On streptozotocin induced diabetic rats. Int Sch Res Notices 2014.
[http://dx.doi.org/10.1155/2014/130342]

[60]   Maruki-Uchida H, Kurita I, Sugiyama K, Sai M, Maeda K, Ito T. The protective effects of piceatannol from passion fruit (*Passiflora edulis*) seeds in UVB-irradiated keratinocytes. Biol Pharm Bull 2013; 36(5): 845-9.
[http://dx.doi.org/10.1248/bpb.b12-00708] [PMID: 23649341]

[61]   Gupta RK, Kumar D, Chaudhary AK, Maithani M, Singh R. Antidiabetic activity of *Passiflora incarnata* Linn. in streptozotocin-induced diabetes in mice. J Ethnopharmacol 2012; 139(3): 801-6.
[http://dx.doi.org/10.1016/j.jep.2011.12.021] [PMID: 22212504]

[62]   Montefusco-Pereira CV, de Carvalho MJ, de Araújo Boleti AP, Teixeira LS, Matos HR, Lima ES. Antioxidant, anti-inflammatory, and hypoglycemic effects of the leaf extract from *Passiflora nitida* Kunth. Appl Biochem Biotechnol 2013; 170(6): 1367-78.
[http://dx.doi.org/10.1007/s12010-013-0271-6] [PMID: 23666642]

[63]   Ichimura T, Yamanaka A, Ichiba T, *et al.* Antihypertensive effect of an extract of *Passiflora edulis* rind in spontaneously hypertensive rats. Biosci Biotechnol Biochem 2006; 70(3): 718-21.
[http://dx.doi.org/10.1271/bbb.70.718] [PMID: 16556991]

[64]   Tommonaro G, Rodríguez CS, Santillana M, *et al.* Chemical composition and biotechnological properties of a polysaccharide from the peels and antioxidative content from the pulp of Passiflora liguralis fruits. J Agric Food Chem 2007; 55(18): 7427-33.
[http://dx.doi.org/10.1021/jf0704615] [PMID: 17676862]

[65]   Zibadi S, Farid R, Moriguchi S, *et al.* Oral administration of purple passion fruit peel extract attenuates blood pressure in female spontaneously hypertensive rats and humans. Nutr Res 2007; 27: 408-16.
[http://dx.doi.org/10.1016/j.nutres.2007.05.004]

[66]   Konta EM, Almeida MR, do Amaral CL, *et al.* Evaluation of the antihypertensive properties of yellow passion fruit pulp (*Passiflora edulis* Sims *f. flavicarpa* Deg.) in spontaneously hypertensive rats. Phytother Res 2014; 28(1): 28-32.
[http://dx.doi.org/10.1002/ptr.4949] [PMID: 23436457]

[67]   Guerrero-Ospina JC, Nieto OA, Zarate MDP, *et al.* Beneficial effects of passiflora edulis on blood pressure and reduction of oxidative stress. Indian J Sci Technol 2018; 11(43): 1-8.
[http://dx.doi.org/10.17485/ijst/2018/v11i43/134064]

[68]   Appel K, Rose T, Fiebich B, Kammler T, Hoffmann C, Weiss G. Modulation of the γ-aminobutyric acid (GABA) system by *Passiflora incarnata* L. Phytother Res 2011; 25(6): 838-43.
[http://dx.doi.org/10.1002/ptr.3352] [PMID: 21089181]

[69]   Patel SS, Verma NK, Shrestha B, Gauthaman K. Antihypertensive effect of methanolic extract of *Passiflora nepalensis.* Braz J Pharmacog 2011; 21(1): 187-9.
[http://dx.doi.org/10.1590/S0102-695X2011005000012]

[70]   Bareño LL, Puebla P, Carlos M. *Passiflora quadrangularis* prevents experimental hypertension and vascular remodelling in rats exposed to nitric oxide deficit. Vitae 2017; 24(3): 186-95.
[http://dx.doi.org/10.17533/udea.vitae.v24n4a04]

CHAPTER 6

Monograph on *Anvillea radiata* Coss. & Durieu

Mourad Akdad and **Mohamed Eddouks**[*]

Team of Ethnopharmacology and Pharmacognosy, Faculty of Sciences and Techniques Errachidia, Moulay Ismail University of Meknes, BP 509, Boutalamine, 52000. Errachidia, Morocco.

Abstract: *Anvillea radiata* Coss. & Durieu (*A. radiata*) which belongs to the Asteraceae family is an aromatic and medicinal plant, endemic of Morocco and Algeria and usually used in the traditional medicines to treat obesity, hypertension and diabetes. The phytochemical analysis of *A. radiata* reveals the presence of a number of bioactive compounds such as germacranolids. The present chapter summarizes the most recent ethnobotanical, pharmacological and phytochemical studies conducted on this herb.

Keywords: *Anvillea Radiate*, Diabetes, Hypertension, Medicinal plant, Phytochemistry, Pharmacology.

INTRODUCTION

Anvillea radiata Coss. & Durieu is a wild plant which belongs to the Asteraceae family (Fig. **1**). This plant is endemic of North Africa (Morocco and Algeria). Based on ethnopharmacological surveys, folkloric practices and phytotherapeutic *A. radiata* as a medicinal plant is used for the treatment of gastroenteritis, spasms, colic, hepatitis, arthritis and rheumatoid, indigestion, lung diseases, obesity and diabetes [1 - 4]. It has been reported to possess many biological effects. This plant showed an antihypertensive effect on L-Name-induced hypertensive rats [5], antihyperglycemic activity in streptozotocin(STZ)-induced diabetic rats [6], and antifungal [8], antitumor [9], and hypolipidemic activities [10] on high-fat diet fed mice [7]. The evaluation of three compounds (two epimergermacranolides, and a phenolic acid) purified from this plant has revealed their potential anticholinesterase and anti-tyrosinase activities, α-glucosidase inhibitory activity, and cytotoxic activity against MCF-7 cancer cell lines [11]. This chapter summarizes traditional uses, phytochemistry and discusses the potential biological activities of *A. radiata*.

---

[*] **Corresponding author Mohamed Eddouks:** Faculty of Sciences and Techniques Errachidia, Moulay Ismail University of Meknes, BP 509, Boutalamine, 52000. Errachidia, Morocco; Tel: +212 5 35 57 44 97; Fax: +212 5 35 57 44 85; E-mail: mohamed.eddouks@laposte.net

Taxonomy and Geographical Location

A. radiata is inherent to North Africa, especially in Morocco and Algeria. It is locally called *Negd, Negdsehraoui, tehetit, nougdl'hoor, Ajri*, and *Gijou* [12 - 15].

The taxonomy of *A. radiata* is as follows:

Kingdom: Plantae

Subkingdom:Tracheobionta

Superdivision: Spermatophyta

Division: Magnoliophyta

Class: Magnoliopsida

Subclass: Asteridae

Order: Asterales

Family: Asteraceae

Genus: Anvillea

Species: radiata

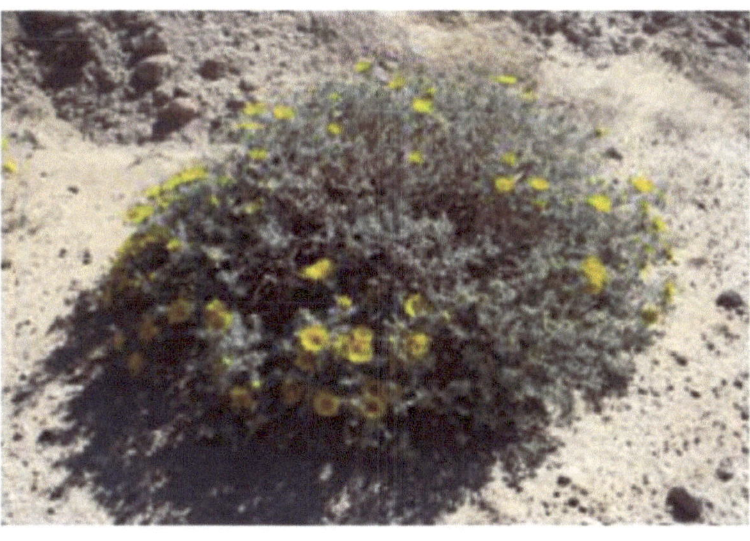

Fig. (1). *Anvillea radiata.*

Use in Traditional Medicine

A. radiata is an endemic plant in Morocco and Algeria. The most common ailments treated with this plant are digestives disorders, affections of glands, infections, pulmonary disorders, and diabetes. Table **1** summarizes the ethnopharmacological uses of *A. radiata* in Morocco and Algeria.

Table 1. Traditional use of *Anvillea radiata*.

Region	Ailments	Parts of Plant	Mode of Preparation	Reference
Morocco	Urinary infections: pyelonephritis pyelonephritis and cystitis	Leaves Leaves	Recipe based on *Anvillea radiata, Origanum compactum, Ricinus communis*, in powder associated with butter, honey and seedless dates is used in the form of suppositories, covered with henna powder and dried in the shade. A recipe based on *Anvillea radiata, Artemisia herba alba, Lavandula dentata, Hyoscyamus albus and Hyoscyamus muticus*, in powder added to *Allium sativum* cooked at steam and dates with no seeds, is used underform suppositories	[14]
	Gastric complaints the cold of the back	Leaves Leaves	The powder The powder of the leaves of *Anvillea radiata* associated with goats' butter is used as suppositories	[13]
	Uro-genital and metabolic disorders; Affections of the glands	Leaves, Whole plant	Infusion, decoction	[15]
	Pathologies of the digestive system, diabetes, Dermocosmotology	Roots, Whole plant	Decoction Oral administration or inhalation	[16 - 18]
	As cholagogue	Flower	Decoction	[19]
Algeria	Diabetes, Indigestion, cold, the stomach aches and the pulmonary diseases	leaves and stems	Maceration, decoction, infusion or inhalation	[20]
	Pulmonary infection, Indigestion	leaves and stems	Infusion, maceration	[21]
	Stomach and liver diseases; Diabetes	aerial parts	Internal use by infusion	[12]

PHYTOCHEMISTRY

Qualitative phytochemical analysis of *A. radiata* aerial parts revealed the presence of polyphenols, flavonoids, tannins, sesquiterpenes, terpenoids, alkaloids, sterols, free quinones, anthraquinones, saponins, emodols, anthracenosides, volatile oils, fatty acids and carbohydrates [6, 8, 22]. Few phytochemical studies have been carried out on this plant so that a group of phytoconstituents such as flavonoids compounds has been found. Thirteen flavonoids were isolated in the MeOH extract of *A. radiata* aerial parts: 4 aglycones (Fig. **2**) and 9 flavonol glycosides (Fig. **3**); these flavonols were mostly glycosylated at the C-3 position, while nine flavonoids were 6-methoxylated [23].

Fig. (2). Flavonoids aglycosides identified in *A radiata*.

Parthenolide and its derivatives (subclass germacranolides) are potent anticancer and anti-inflammatory molecules [24, 25]. Many studies have been focused on this phytocompounds because of their abilities to target specific signaling pathways or molecules in cancer [26]. Parthenolide was identified for the first time in *Tanacetum parthenium* mainly in the plant shoots, or aerial parts (flowers and leaves) [27, 28]. Meanwhile, the total synthesis of parthenolide is so difficult regarding the complexity of its skeleton and the presence of many chiral centers [29]. Commercially available parthenolide has been extracted from the leaves of *Chrysanthemum parthenium* (Enzo Life Sciences and Cayman Chemical) [26]. However, it is difficult to purify the natural form of this compound in order to develop a new pharmaceutical or adjuvant in the treatment of cancer and inflammation and further hemi-synthesis. In this context, *A. radiata* is a promising source of germacranolides. The most common compounds identified in *A. radiata* are germacranolides, which are present in high amounts in addition to flavonoids.

However, the separation of both classes of compounds is a constraint to obtain high amounts of parthenolides. Maceration, liquid-liquid extraction, and silica gel column chromatography have been exploited to isolate germacranolides from chloroform extracts of the aerial parts of *A. radiata*, but they afforded to isolate only a small amount [29]. Centrifugal Partition Chromatography (CPC), allows the separation and purification of several phytocompounds, and has been used by Destandau *et al.*, (2015) to isolate molecules from *A. radiata*. CPC is a technique allowing the separation of compounds through a column by the use of two non-miscible liquids [29]. Preliminary, HPLC-ELSD technique which is used to detect molecules without any chromophore group, showed two pics corresponding to germacranolide, despite the HPLC-UV technique considered as more sensitive for the flavonoids [29]. On the other hand, authors have demonstrated that the CPC technique was able to separate germacranolides and flavonoids and the two hydroxyparthenolides 9-α and 9-β with purity over 99% [29]. The most cited germacranolides identified in aerial parts of *A. radiata* are 9α-hydroxyparthenolide, parthenolid-9-one and 8α,9α-epoxyparthenolide. These compounds contain the same 4α,5β-epoxygermacrene-6α,7β-olide skeleton (Table 2) [30].

Fig. 3 cont.....

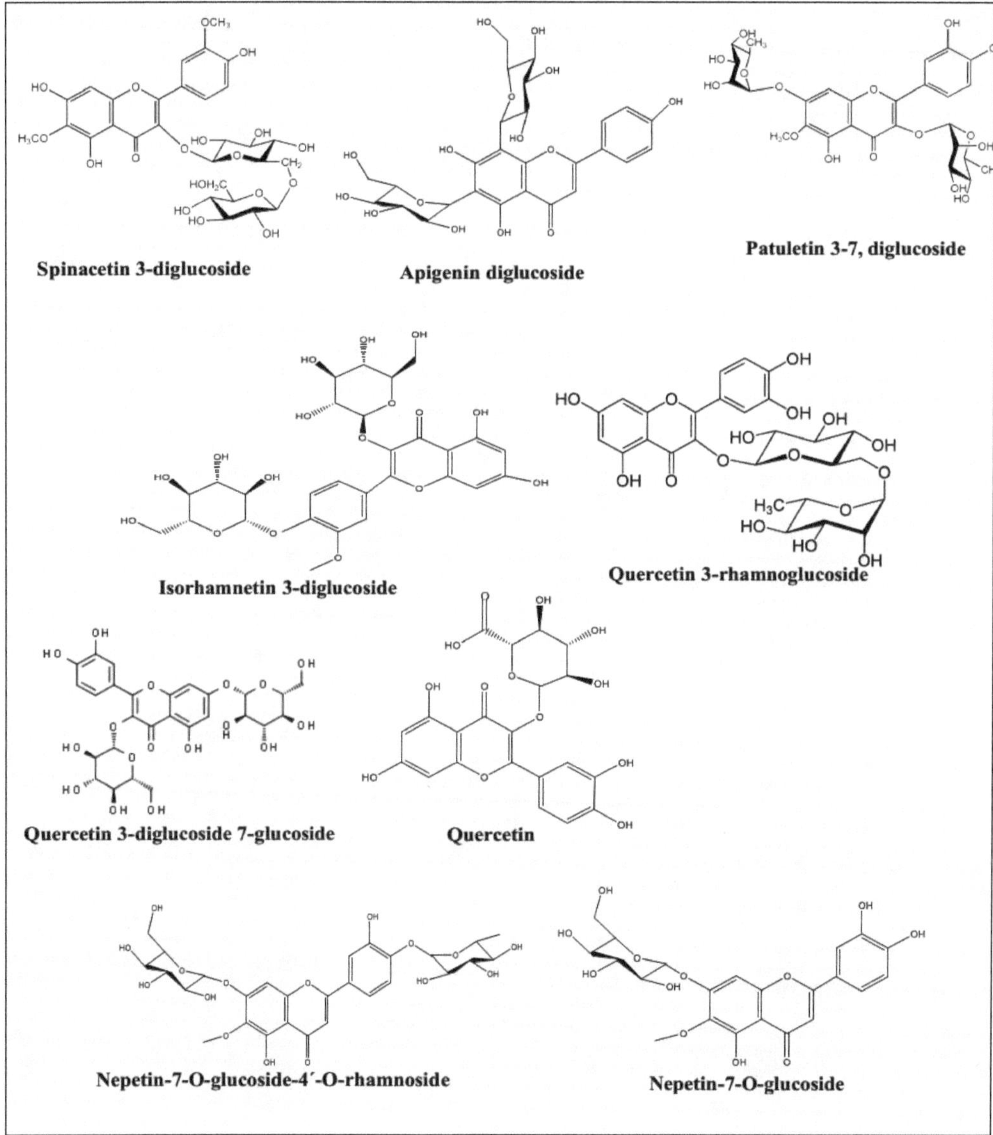

Fig. (3). Glycosides identified in *A radiata*.

In another study, using Accelerated Solvent Extraction (ASE) in two steps, Boukhris *et al*, (2016) successfully isolated flavonoids and germacranolides from aerial parts of *A. radiata*. This technique, also known as pressurized liquid extraction, has been used to analyze molecules present in a low amount in the environment, plant, or nutrition [31]. Firstly, using chloroform as a solvent, germacranolides were removed and then, by methanol phenolic compounds were extracted and characterized. Phenolics profile revealed the presence of chlorogenic acid and dicaffeoylquinic acid derivatives and both flavonoids aglycones and glycosides [32]. Then, the phytochemical composition of the whole plant was compared with each organ (flower, leave and stem). The stem and leaves had the same profile, but not the flowers. The same compounds identified in the aerial parts were also found in the organs, while a difference in concentration was noted. Flowers contain di-caffeoylquinic acid derivative as the most abundant compound, while stems and leaves contain isorhamnetin and spinacitindiglucoside derivatives [32]. In our report on the phytochemical analysis of *A. radiata* aerial parts, we showed that chlorogenic acid is the most abundant phenolic in the ethanol extract with a concentration of 214.18 mg/kg. Caffeoylquinate isomers, caffeic, and chlorogenic acids were also identified. Besides, the flavonoids quercetinglucuronide, nepetin-7-O-glucoside-4′-O-rhamnoside, and apigenindiglucoside were reported for the first time in this species [5]. Figs. (**2-6**) summarize the known phytochemical components of *A. radiata*.

Fig. (4). Germacranolides identified in *A radiata.*

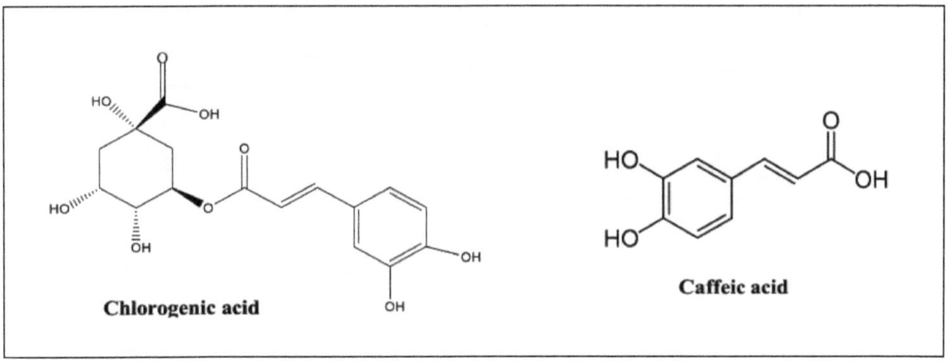

Chlorogenic acid

Caffeic acid

Fig. (5). Hydroxycinnamic derivatives identified in *A radiata*.

Di-O-caffeoylquinic Acid

3,5-Dicaffeoylquinic

eruloyl-caffeoylquinic acid

Diferuloylquinic acid

Neochlorogenic acid

Cryptochlorogenic acid

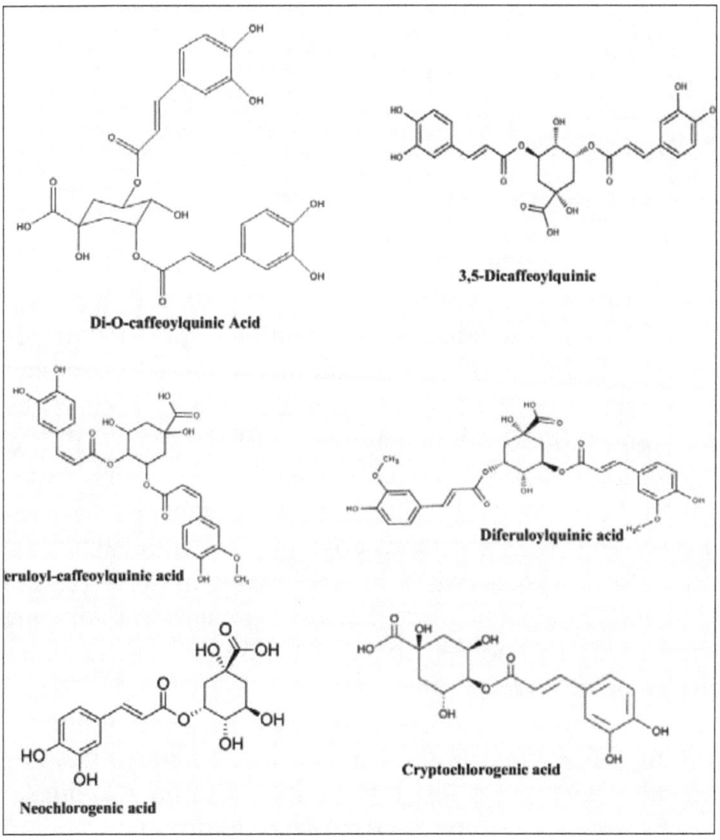

Fig. 6. Quinic acids and derivatives class identified in *A radiata*.

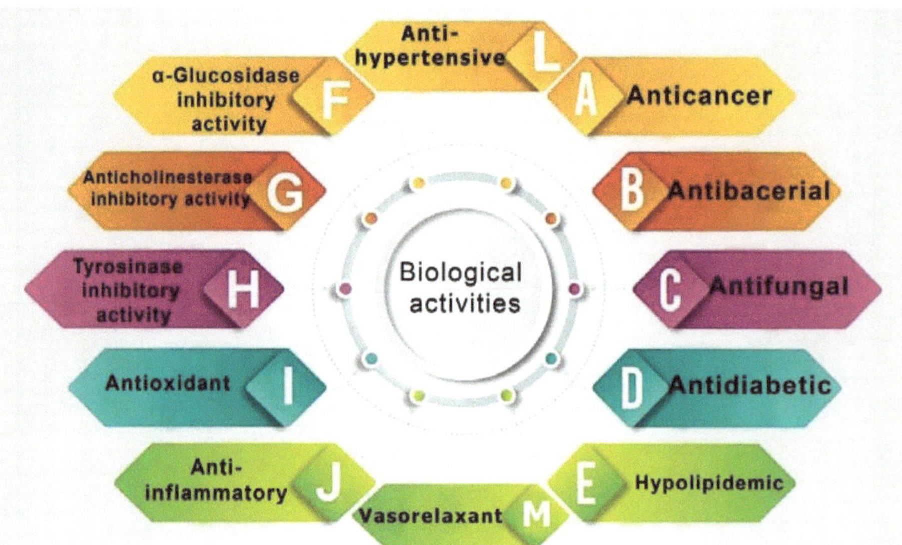

Fig. (7). The main biological activities of *A radiata.*

ANTIOXIDANT ACTIVITY

A. radiata has been demonstrated to exhibit some biological activities (Fig. **7**). Several *in vitro* experiments showed that *A. radiata* possesses a potent antioxidant capacity [33 - 36]. The study conducted by Saoud *et al.*, (2019) has demonstrated that *A radiata* EtOAc extract is more puissant to scavenge free radical than the n-BuOH. The EtOAc and n-BuOH extracts have a strong antioxidant capacity with an IC_{50} of 0.0034 and 0.0026 mg/mL against DPPH radical (IC_{50} of BHT was 0.018 mg/mL), while it was 0.002 to 0.001 mg/mL for the ABTS assay (IC_{50} of BHT was 0.05 mg/ml), respectively. The antioxidant capacity of medicinal plants is known to be correlated with phenolics content. The high capacity of *A radiata* EtOAc to scavenge free radicals than n-butanol extract may be related to the high amount of total phenolic detected when the two extracts were compared by Folin-Ciocalteu method [11]. In another study, Kandouli *et al*, (2017) studied the antioxidant activity of *A. radiata* polar and nonpolar extracts against a series of determinants of ROS (inhibition of Cu^{2+}-induced LDL oxidation, HO scavenging activity, inhibition of deoxyribose degradation, metal chelating capacity, Superoxide radical scavenging (O2) capacity, Xanthine oxidase inhibition, Oxygen radical absorbing capacity, total reactive antioxidant potential and 2,2-Diphenyl-1-picrylhydrazyl (DPPH) radical scavenging assays). In the DPPH assay, all the extracts (methanol, petroleum ether, ethyl acetate, butanol, aqueous residual fraction, lyophilized aqueous extracts) showed free radical reducing activity with different kinetics behavior and capacities. The highest inhibition was obtained with ethyl acetate and butanol extracts with IC_{50} values of 43.5±0.1 and 47.9±2.6 µg/mL, respectively. Consistently, in ORAC and TRAP assays the potent scavenging of peroxyl radicals was obtained for the ethyl acetate and butanol extracts [7]. In addition, the XO inhibition test by measuring uric acid production revealed weak XO inhibitory activities of all extracts when compared with allopurinol and quercetin. In contrast, in O_2 scavenging test appreciable inhibition was noted as detected by low IC50 values (<0.3 µg/mL), and in ferrozine assay extracts revealed a moderate activity in comparison to the positive control with strong variation among extracts and the highest inhibition was demonstrated for PE extract (70.9±9.2 µmol EDTAE/g) [7].

On the hemolysis test measuring free radical-induced erythrocyte lysis in whole blood and its inhibition by antioxidants, *A. radiata* hydromethanolic extract has demonstrated a beneficial effect against free radical damage in addition to a good free radical (DPPH) scavenging activity with an EC_{50} of 21.73±0.09 mg/L [37]. *A. radiata* has shown potent antioxidant activity against different ROS and inhibited or reversed damages induced by oxidative stress, suggesting that this plant could be used as a source of natural antioxidants in food supplements or in the pharmaceutical industry.

ANTIDIABETIC AND HYPOLIPIDEMIC ACTIVITIES

In streptozotocin(STZ)-induced diabetic rats, the aqueous extract of *A. radiata* leaves provoked a potent antihyperglycemic activity in the acute and sub-chronic studies. Single oral administration of *A. radiata* at a dose of 10 mg/kg reduced plasma glucose level after six hours of the treatment (p<0.0001). Additionally, daily oral administration of *A. radiata* aqueous extract to STZ rats for fifteen days normalized the blood glucose at the end of the study (p<0.0001). Moreover, *A. radiata* reversed the pancreatic and hepatic histopathological damages induced by STZ. In glucose tolerance test, *A. radiata* prevented the increase in the blood glucose levels after treatment by glucose suggesting that increase of insulin secretion, inhibition of α-amylase and α-glucosidase and/or increase glucose uptake by adipocyte and skeletal muscle are possible mechanisms of action by which *A. radiata* reduce blood glucose in diabetic rats [6]. The presence of tannins and flavonoids in medicinal and aromatic plants was reported to be responsible for the anti-diabetic effect [38, 39]. The phytochemical analysis of *A. radiata* revealed the presence of several secondary metabolites such as tannins and flavonoids with potent antioxidant capacity [10]. Free radical scavenging activity may be responsible for the observed effect that inhibits STZ-induced free radicals damage of β cell. In accordance, another study showed that *A. radiata* ameliorated glycemia in type 2 diabetes [7]. In high-fat fed C57/BL6J mice, different doses of *A. radiata* n-butanol and aqueous extracts (25, 75, 150 and 250 mg/kg) showed blood glucose-lowering activity after 4h from the treatment, with a maximum reduction at a dose of 150 mg/kg. In addition, 16 weeks of treatment of mice showed a significant antihyperglycemic, antihyperlipidemic and anti-inflammatory activity, and delayed oxidative stress-induced myocardial and muscle damage [7]. Several studies have focused their works on the inhibition of carbohydrate-hydrolyzing enzymes by medicinal and aromatic plants to manage postprandial blood glucose levels of type 2 diabetics. The most targeted enzymes are α-amylase and α-glucosidase [40, 41]. *A. radiata* possesses an antidiabetic effect *in vitro*. EtOAc and BuOH extracts are able to inhibit α-glucosidase activity [11]. EtOAc and BuOH extracts have demonstrated the same inhibitory activity with an IC_{50} of 0.92 and 0.81 mg/ml respectively, whereas the positive control acarbose inhibits α-glucosidase activity with an IC_{50} of 0.07 mg/ml. This capacity may be helpful to reduce postprandial glucose levels [11]. In addition, *A. radiata* ameliorated lipidic status of normal and STZ rats. Fifteen days of daily oral administration of *A. radiata* aqueous extract (10 mg/kg) decreased TG, and TC with a significant increase of HDL-C in both normal and diabetics rats [10]. However, the antidiabetic effect of *A. radiata* possibly involved modulation of oxidative status [6, 7], inhibition of carbohydrate-hydrolyzing enzymes [7, 11], attenuation of inflammation [7], enhancement of lipidic profiles by decreasing the bad cholesterols and increasing good cholesterol [7, 10]. Generally, *A. radiata* is considered as a promising source to develop neutraceutical for the management of diabetes mellitus.

ANTIMICROBIAL ACTIVITY

In vitro studies have conducted to evaluate the antimicrobial activity of *A. radiata*. Many bacterial strains are sensible to *A. radiata* or molecules isolated from this plant such as Gram-negative strains: *Klebseilla pneumonie* (ATCC700603), *Pseudomonas aeriginosa* (ATCC 9721), *Escherichia coli* (ATCC 25922), *Escherichia coli* (ATCC 8739) and *Salmonella abony* (NCTC 6017) and Gram-positive strains: *Staphylococcus aureus* (ATCC25923), *Streptocoque*, *Staphylococcus aureus* (ATCC 29213), *Staphylococcus aureus* (ATCC 6538) and *Bacillus subtilis* (ATCC 6633) [11, 22, 30, 42, 43]. Methanolic extract of *A. radiata* has revealed a potent antibacterial effect against Gram-positive strains: *Staphylococcus aureus* and *Streptocoque* (MIC of 150 and 75 µg/ml, respectively) [22]. However, the aqueous extract of *A. radiata* leaves has shown strong antibacterial activity against multidrug-resistant strains. The highest antibacterial effect of *A. radiata* was noted against *Escherichia coli* with a MIC of 12.5 mg/ml [42]. In a comparative study of antimicrobial activity of the aqueous, methanolic and ethyl acetate *A. radiata* extracts showed a promising antimicrobial effect and the methanolic extract showed the strong inhibitory effect on bacterial growth against the Gram-negative Salmonella abony (NCTC 6017) with a MIC value of

0.42 mg/ml [43]. In another study, using the microdilution method, Saoud *et al.*, (2019) have demonstrated that EtOAc and BuOH extracts were active against Gram-positive and Gram-negative bacteria with MIC values ranging from 0.062 to 0.250 mg/m. However, when compared with the positive control vancomycin (MIC 0.001 to 0.004 mg/mL) the antibacterial effect exerted by these extracts was very limited. Contrariwise, when isolated compounds from *A. radiata* were tested alone (9α-hydroxyparthenolide, 9β-hydroxyparthenolide or 3,5-O-dicaffeoylquinic acid) to inhibit the growth of the same panel of bacteria, antibacterial activity was more puissant (MIC varied from 0.015 to 0.125 mg/mL). The authors suggested an antagonism effect between the different compounds present as an explanation of the observed effect [11]. On the other side, 9α-hydroxyparthenolide isolated from aerial parts of *A. radiata* inhibited the growth of *Bacillus cereus, Streptococcus C, Enterococcus faecalis, Escherichia coli,* and *Proteus vulgaris* at concentrations of 50 and 100 µg/disc [30].

ANTIFUNGAL ACTIVITY

A study conducted by Askarne *et al.*, (2012) screened eight medicinal and aromatic plants from Morocco and evaluated their extracts with different types of solvents for antifungal activity against *Penicillium italicum* [44]. The authors have shown that chloroformic extracts of *A. radiata* leaves and stem possess the highest antifungal activity against the citrus blue mould with a MIC value of 2 mg/ml. On the other hand, *in vivo* treatment of citrus fruits by chloroformic extract of *A. radiata* for 2h before pathogen inoculation revealed a decrease in the incidence and severity of the blue mould, after 7 and 10 days of storage at 20°C in comparison to the control untreated fruits. *A. radiata* may be an alternative to chemical fungicides against major postharvest citrus fungal pathogens [45]. "*Bayoud* disease" is the biggest threat of date palm worldwide. Pathogenic fungi *Fusarium oxysporum f. sp. albedinis* (Foa) is the causal agent of this disease. *In vitro* and *in vivo* investigations have been performed to search new drugs from medicinal and aromatic plants to prevent and/or treat *Bayoud* disease. Mebarki *et al*, (2013) evaluated the antifungal activity of flavonoid and cell-wall polysaccharide extracts from leaves and flowers of *A. radiata* against Foa. The authors demonstrated that on spore germination assay, at all dosages used (0.25-4 mg/ml), flavonoid extracts from leaves or flowers inhibited spore germination with a percentage of spore germination varying from 70 to 42.83% (while the percentage in control was 83.44%). On mycelial growth, hemicellulose, highly methylated pectins (HMP) or flavonoid extracts induced an inhibitory activity in a dose-dependent manner (0.5-4 mg/ml). HMP from flowers have shown the strongest inhibition of mycelial growth fungal strain colony radius 3.18 cm (4.59 cm in the control) [8].

ANTICANCER ACTIVITY

9α-hydroxyparthenolide isolated from aerial parts of *A. radiata* showed significant cytotoxic activity against five human cancer cell lines, with an IC_{50} of 2 µg/ml against A 549, H 116, PSN 1 and SKBR 3 and IC_{50}>5 µg/ml against T98G [30]. Currently, 9-hydroxyamino-parthenolides synthesized by amination of germacranolids isolated from *A. radiata* revealed a potent anticancer activity against murine and human cancer cell lines [46]. 9α- and 9β-hydroxyparthenolide isolated from the aerial parts of *A. radiata* were subject to Heck or Acylation reactions at the C-9 and C-13 positions in order to evaluate their *in vitro* anticancer activity. Among the twenty-one synthetic compounds from parthenolides of *A. radiata*, seven have shown a potent anticancer activity (IC50 values ranging from 1.1 to 9.4 µM) against HS-683, SK-MEL-28, A549, and MCF-7 human cancer cell lines. Authors have demonstrated that methylene--lactone moiety free at the C13 position of 9α-hydroxyparthenolide isolated from *A. radiata* is necessary for its anticancer activity because when it is modified the cytotoxicity was decreased [47].

ANTIHYPERTENSIVE ACTIVITY

Medicinal plants have received a great deal of attention in the management of hypertension. *In vivo* and clinical studies have demonstrated that aromatic plants are a promising source to develop new antihypertensive drugs. The plant *A. radiata* exhibited antihypertensive activity in L-Name-induced hypertensive rats [5]. This study has been carried out using *in vivo* and *in vitro* investigations. In *in vivo* experiments, in normotensive and L-Name-induced hypertensive rats single and daily oral administration for seven days at a dose of 100 mg/kg of *A. radiata* aqueous extract were evaluated by monitoring systolic blood pressure (SBP), mean blood pressure (MBP), diastolic blood pressure (DBP), and heart rate (HR). Using *ex vivo* vascular reactivity assays, we assessed the vasorelaxant activity of *A. radiata* aqueous extract (0.08-0.64 mg/ml) in thoracic aortic rings pre-contracted by Epinephrine (10 µM) or KCl (80 mM). The results of our study revealed that a single administration of *A. radiata* provoked a rapid decrease in arterial blood pressure of hypertensive rats without affecting the heart rate. The aqueous extract of *A. radiata* showed a potent antihypertensive effect on hypertensive rats during seven days of treatment. This antihypertensive effect of *A. radiata* was comparable to the standard drug Lasilix at 20 mg/kg. In contrast, no significant effect was noted in normotensive rats treated. In addition, *in vitro* investigation has shown that *A. radiata* aqueous extract (0.08-0.64 mg/ml) induced vasorelaxant activity in a dose-dependent manner in blood vessels pre-contracted by EP or KCl, suggesting that vasodilatation is one of the mechanisms by which *A. radiata* induced antihypertensive activity. To explore the mechanism underlying the vasorelaxant effect of *A. radiata*, pre-incubation for 20 min of the isolated aortic ring with Nifidepine, Methylene blue, Indomethacin, Glibenclamide, Propranolol, or L-Name has been conducted before EP-evoked contraction. The vasorelaxant effect induced by *A. radiata* was abrogated when the aortic rings were pre-incubated with Nifidepine, L-NAME, or Methylene blue, indicating that inhibition of Ca^{2+} entry through calcium channels, direct NO and NO-cGMP pathways are involved in the vasorelaxant activity of *A. radiata* [5]. On the other side, we analyzed the phytochemical profile of *A. radiata* by analytical HPLC and HPLC-ESI-MS to characterize the main bioactive compounds present in this herb. We identified different types of secondary metabolites such as caffeoylquinic acids, chlorogenic and caffeic acids based on their retention times, UV absorbance, authentic standards, and mass spectra, as well as by comparison with literature data [5]. The effect of isolated caffeoylquinic acids on SBP on spontaneously hypertensive rats was evaluated by Mishima *et al*, (2005). The authors demonstrated that a single oral administration of 3,5-diCQA at a dose of 10 mg/kg/10 ml induced a significant reduction of systolic blood pressure, without affecting heart rate [48]. Another study showed that single oral administration of chlorogenic acid (30–300 mg/kg) reduced the systolic blood pressure of spontaneously hypertensive rats in a dose-dependent manner. The chronic evaluation of the chlorogenic acid effect on arterial blood pressure revealed that treatment for 8 weeks at a dose of 300 mg/kg per day inhibited the development of hypertension on spontaneously hypertensive rats. Besides, chlorogenic acid was able to ameliorate endothelial function [49]. The evaluation of chlorogenic and caffeic acids' cardiovascular effect on cyclosporine-induced hypertensive rats has shown that chlorogenic and caffeic acids normalized arterial blood pressure. This effect was accompanied by inhibition of acetylcholinesterase, butrylcholinesterase and arginase activities, improvement of nitric oxide bioavailability and antioxidant status suggesting that chlorogenic and caffeic acids act at a different level to improve hypertensive status provoked by cyclosporine [50]. In human hypertensive subjects, four weeks of treatment by chlorogenic acid at a dose of 25 mg/kg per day decreased blood pressure [51]. Consequently, 3,5-di-caffeoylquinic acid, and chlorogenic and caffeic acids could account for the antihypertensive activity of *A. radiata* observed in our study.

ANTICHOLINESTERASE ACTIVITY

In the central and peripheral nervous systems, Acetylcholinesterase (AChE) has a crucial role in hydrolyzing acetylcholine, leading to the breakdown of acetylcholine [52]. This reduction of acetylcholine concentration can be prevented by the inhibition of AChE [53]. Recently, the development of new potent AChE inhibitors from natural products is getting attention and several classes of secondary metabolites have shown this ability such as alkaloids [54], phenolic compounds [55], and terpenes [56]. *A. radiata* EtOAc extract inhibited cholinesterase enzyme with an IC_{50} of 0.071 mg/mL [11] suggesting that this herb may be helpful to the patient suffering from Alzheimer's disease.

TYROSINASE INHIBITORY ACTIVITY

A. radiata possesses a Tyrosinase inhibitory activity. EtOAc and BuOH extracts have demonstrated a potent Tyrosinase inhibitory activity when compared to Hydroquinone used as a positive control, the percentage of inhibition was 68.05% and 41.23%, for both EtOAc and BuOH extracts, respectively, while it was 72% for Hydroquinone [11]. Tyrosinase is known as a key enzyme in the mammalian melanogenesis and the melanin produced is very important to protect skin against ultraviolet damage [57]. In contrast, the overproduction of melanin is an esthetic problem because of the more pigmented patches [58].

Table 2. Main active phytochemical compounds isolated from the aerial parts of *A. radiata* from Morocco and Algeria.

Compound	Formula	Structure	Activity	Reference
9α-hydroxyparthenolide	$C_{15}H_{20}O_4$	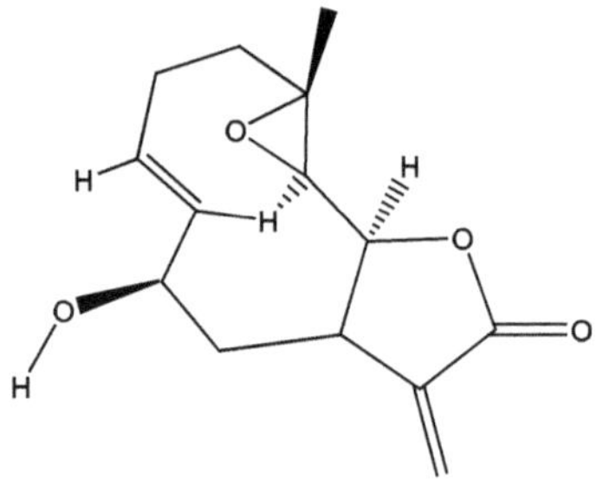	-Cytotoxic activity against A 549, H 116, PSN 1, T98G and SKBR 3. - Inhibited the growth of Bacillus cereus, *Streptococcus C, Enterococcus faecalis, Escherichia coli,* and *Proteus vulgaris* -α-Glucosidase inhibitory activity -Anticholinesterase inhibitory activity -Tyrosinase inhibitory activity	[30]
9β-hydroxyparthenolide.	$C_{15}H_{20}O_4$	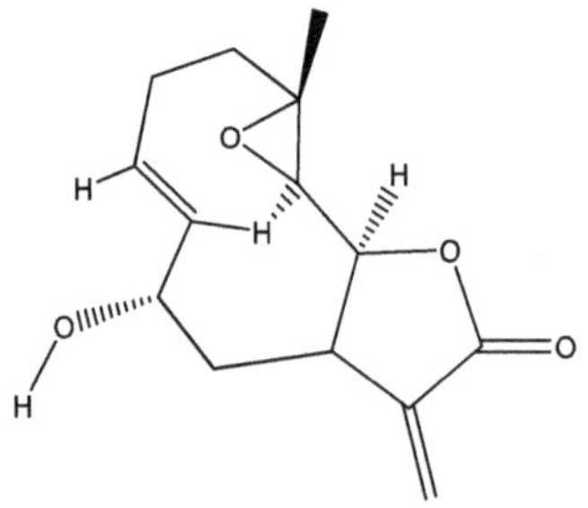	-α-Glucosidase inhibitory activity -Anticholinesterase inhibitory activity -Tyrosinase inhibitory activity -Antibacterial and antifungal -Cytotoxic	[11]

(Table 2) cont.....

Compound	Formula	Structure	Activity	Reference
3,5-O-dicaffeoylquinic acid	$C_{25}H_{24}O_{12}$		- α-Glucosidase inhibitory activity -Anticholinesterase inhibitory activity -Tyrosinase inhibitory -Antibacterial, antifungal and cytotoxic activities	[11]

CONCLUSION

This chapter summarizes the main pharmacological activities of *A. radiata* including antidiabetic, antihypertensive, hypolipidemic, antioxidant, antibacterial, antifungal, and anti-inflammatory effects. Moreover, the phytochemical studies showed clearly that the main constituents of *A. radiata* are germacranolides that have a potent cytotoxic compound against human cancer cell lines. The folkloric practice of Algerian and Moroccan populations revealed that this medicinal plant is mostly used for the treatment of digestive disorders, hepatitis, arthritis, rheumatoid, lung diseases, obesity and diabetes. Both beneficial effects investigated pharmacologically and the richness of this plant on bioactive molecules justify and support the use of this plant for human healthcare from ancient times. On the other hand, the mechanisms of action involved in the cited pharmacological activities of *A. radiata* are still unclear, so future studies are necessary and clinical trials are needed to demonstrate these activities on humans with regard to the safety of this herb.

FUNDING

This study was supported by Centre National pour la Recherche Scientifique et Technique (CNRST) (Grant Number PPR/2015/35).

CONSENT FOR PUBLICATION

Not applicable.

CONFLICT OF INTEREST

There is no conflict of interest declared.

ACKNOWLEDGEMENT

Declared none.

REFERENCES

[1]   Eddouks M, Ajebli M, Hebi M. Ethnopharmacological survey of medicinal plants used in Daraa-Tafilalet region (Province of Errachidia), Morocco. J Ethnopharmacol 2017; 198: 516-30.
[http://dx.doi.org/10.1016/j.jep.2016.12.017] [PMID: 28003130]

[2]   Farid O, Khallouki F, Akdad M, Breuer A, Owen RW, Eddouks M. Phytochemical characterization of polyphenolic compounds with HPLC-DAD-ESI-MS and evaluation of lipid-lowering capacity of aqueous extracts from Saharan plant *Anabasis aretioides* (Coss & Moq.) in normal and streptozotocin-induced diabetic rats. J Integr Med 2018; 16(3): 185-91.
[http://dx.doi.org/10.1016/j.joim.2018.03.003] [PMID: 29631911]

[3]   Bellakhdar J. The traditional Moroccan Pharmacopea Ancient Arabic medicine and popular knowledge. Paris: Ibis Press 1997.

[4]   Telli A, Esnault MA, Khelil AO. An ethnopharmacological survey of plants used in traditional diabetes treatment in southeastern Algeria (Ouargla province). J Arid Environ 2016; 127: 82-92.
[http://dx.doi.org/10.1016/j.jaridenv.2015.11.005]

[5]   Akdad M, Ajebli M, Breuer A, Khallouki F, Owen RW, Eddouks M. Study of antihypertensive activity of *Anvillea radiata* in L-NAME-induced hypertensive rats and HPLC-ESI-MS analysis. Endocr Metab Immune Disord Drug Targets 2019; 19: 1.
[http://dx.doi.org/10.2174/1871530319666191115114023] [PMID: 31729295]

[6]   Hebi M, Eddouks M. Glucose Lowering Activity of *Anvillea Radiata* Coss & Durieu in Diabetic Rats. Cardiovasc Hematol Disord Drug Targets 2018; 18(1): 71-80.
[http://dx.doi.org/10.2174/1871529X18666180223100427] [PMID: 29473527]

[7]   Kandouli C, Cassien M, Mercier A, *et al.* Antidiabetic, antioxidant and anti inflammatory properties of water and n-butanol soluble extracts from Saharian *Anvillea radiata* in high-fat-diet fed mice. J Ethnopharmacol 2017; 207: 251-67.
[http://dx.doi.org/10.1016/j.jep.2017.06.042] [PMID: 28669771]

[8]   Mebarki L. KaidHarche M, Benlarbi L, Rahmani A, Sarhani A. Phytochemicalanalysis and antifungal activity of *Anvillea radiata*. World Appl Sci J 2013; 26(2): 165-71.

[9]   Abdel Sattar E, Galal AM, Mossa GS. Antitumor germacranolides from *Antitumor germacranolides*. J Nat Prod 1996; 59(4): 403-5.
[http://dx.doi.org/10.1021/np960064g] [PMID: 8699183]

[10]   Hebi M, Eddouks M. Study of Hypolipidemic and Antioxidant Activities of *Anvillea radiata* Coss & Durieu in Diabetic Rats. Immunol Endocr Metab Agents Med Chem 2017; 17(2): 140-8.
[http://dx.doi.org/10.2174/1871522218666180319163700]

[11]   Saoud DH, Jelassi A, Hlila MB, Goudjil MB, Ladjel S, Ben Jannet H. Biological activities of extracts and metabolites isolated from *Anvillea radiata* Coss. & Dur. (Asteraceae). S Afr J Bot 2019; 121: 386-93.
[http://dx.doi.org/10.1016/j.sajb.2018.10.033]

[12]   Hammiche V, Maiza K. Traditional medicine in Central Sahara: pharmacopoeia of Tassili N'ajjer. J Ethnopharmacol 2006; 105(3): 358-67.
[http://dx.doi.org/10.1016/j.jep.2005.11.028] [PMID: 16414225]

[13]   Ghourri M, Zidane L, El Yacoubi H, Rochdi A, Fadli M, Douira A. Etude floristique et ethnobotanique des plantes médicinales de la ville d'El Ouatia (Maroc Saharien). Kastamonu Univ. Journal of Forestry Faculty 2012; 12(2): 218-35.

[14]   Ghourri M, Zidane L, Douira A. La phytothérapie et les infections urinaires (La pyélonéphrite et la cystite) au Sahara Marocain (Tan-Tan). J Anim Plant Sci 2014; 20(3): 3171-93.

[15]   Bammou M, Daoudi A, Sellam K. El rhaffari L, Ibijbijen J, Nassiri L. Étude Ethnobotanique des Astéracées dans la Région Meknès-Tafilalet (Maroc). International Journal of Innovation and Applied Studies 2015; 13(4): 789-815.

[16]   Fact sheet N134 2008.http://www.who.int/mediacentre/factsheets/2003/fs134/en/

[17]   Mahomoodally MF. Traditional medicines in Africa: an appraisal of ten potent african medicinal plants. Evid Based Complement Alternat Med 2013; 2013617459
[http://dx.doi.org/10.1155/2013/617459] [PMID: 24367388]

[18]   Jamila F, Mostafa E. Ethnobotanical survey of medicinal plants used by people in Oriental Morocco to manage various ailments. J Ethnopharmacol 2014; 154(1): 76-87.
[http://dx.doi.org/10.1016/j.jep.2014.03.016] [PMID: 24685583]

[19]   Merzouki A, Ed-derfoufi F, Molero Mesa J. Contribution to the knowledge of Rifian traditional medicine. II: Folk medicine in Ksar Lakbir district (NW Morocco). Fitoterapia 2000; 71(3): 278-307.
[http://dx.doi.org/10.1016/S0367-326X(00)00139-8] [PMID: 10844168]

[20]   Djellouli M, Moussaoui A, Benmehdi H, *et al.* Ethnopharmacological study and phytochemical screening of three plants (Asteraceae family) from the region of south West Algeria. Asian Journal of Natural &Applied Sciences 2013; 2(2): 59-65.

[21]   hadj MD Ould el , M Hadj-mahammed , H Zabeirou , A. Chehma . importance des plantes spontanées médicinales dans la pharmacopée traditionnelle de la région de Ouargla (Sahara septentrional - Est algérien) Sciences & Technologie 2003; (20): 73-8.

[22]   Hamada D, Ladjel S. Chemical Composition, In-Vitro Anti-microbial and Antioxidant Activities of the Methanolic Extract of *Anvillea radiata* Asteraceae. Res J Pharm Biol Chem Sci 2015; 6(2): 1367-73.

[23]   Dendougui H, Jay M, Benayache F, Benayache S. Flavonoids from *Anvillea radiata* Coss. & Dur. (Asteraceae). Biochem Syst Ecol 2006; 34(9): 718-20.
[http://dx.doi.org/10.1016/j.bse.2006.05.002]

[24]   Wiedhopf RM, Young M, Bianchi E, Cole JR. Tumor inhibitory agent from Magnolia grandiflora (Magnoliaceae). I. Parthenolide. J Pharm Sci 1973; 62(2): 345.
[http://dx.doi.org/10.1002/jps.2600620244] [PMID: 4686424]

[25]   Bork PM, Schmitz ML, Kuhnt M, Escher C, Heinrich M. Sesquiterpene lactone containing Mexican Indian medicinal plants and pure sesquiterpene lactones as potent inhibitors of transcription factor NF-kappaB. FEBS Lett 1997; 402(1): 85-90.
[http://dx.doi.org/10.1016/S0014-5793(96)01502-5] [PMID: 9013864]

[26]   Ghantous A, Sinjab A, Herceg Z, Darwiche N. Parthenolide: from plant shoots to cancer roots. Drug Discov Today 2013; 18(17-18): 894-905.
[http://dx.doi.org/10.1016/j.drudis.2013.05.005] [PMID: 23688583]

[27]   Bohlmann F, Zdero C. Sesquiterpene lactones and other constituents from Tanacetumparthenium. Phytochemistry 1982; 21(10): 2543-9.
[http://dx.doi.org/10.1016/0031-9422(82)85253-9]

[28]   Stojakowska A, Kisiel W. Production of parthenolide in organ cultures of feverfew. Plant Cell Tissue Organ Cult 1997; 47: 159-62.
[http://dx.doi.org/10.1007/BF02318952]

[29]   Destandau E, Boukhris MA, Zubrzycki S, Akssira M, Rhaffari LE, Elfakir C. Centrifugal partition chromatography elution gradient for isolation of sesquiterpene lactones and flavonoids from *Anvillea radiata.* J Chromatogr B Analyt Technol Biomed Life Sci 2015; 985: 29-37.
[http://dx.doi.org/10.1016/j.jchromb.2015.01.019] [PMID: 25647341]

[30]   El Hassany B, El Hanbali F, Akssira M, Mellouki F, Haidour A, Barrero AF. Germacranolides from *Anvillea radiata.* Fitoterapia 2004; 75(6): 573-6.
[http://dx.doi.org/10.1016/j.fitote.2004.06.003] [PMID: 15351111]

[31]   Sun H, Ge X, Lv Y, Wang A. Application of accelerated solvent extraction in the analysis of organic contaminants, bioactive and nutritional compounds in food and feed. J Chromatogr A 2012; 1237: 1-

23.
[http://dx.doi.org/10.1016/j.chroma.2012.03.003] [PMID: 22465684]

[32]   Alaoui Boukhris M, Destandau E, El Hakmaoui A, El Rhaffari L, Elfakir C. A dereplication strategy for the identification of new phenolic compounds from *Anvillea radiata* (Coss. &Durieu). C R Chim 2016; 19(9): 1124-32.
[http://dx.doi.org/10.1016/j.crci.2016.05.019]

[33]   Rajendran P, Nandakumar N, Rengarajan T, *et al.* Antioxidants and human diseases. Clin Chim Acta 2014; 436: 332-47.
[http://dx.doi.org/10.1016/j.cca.2014.06.004] [PMID: 24933428]

[34]   Wu JQ, Kosten TR, Zhang XY. Free radicals, antioxidant defense systems, and schizophrenia. Prog Neuropsychopharmacol Biol Psychiatry 2013; 46: 200-6.
[http://dx.doi.org/10.1016/j.pnpbp.2013.02.015] [PMID: 23470289]

[35]   Taniyama Y, Griendling KK. Reactive oxygen species in the vasculature: molecular and cellular mechanisms. Hypertension 2003; 42(6): 1075-81.
[http://dx.doi.org/10.1161/01.HYP.0000100443.09293.4F] [PMID: 14581295]

[36]   Pizzino G, Irrera N, Cucinotta M, *et al.* Oxidative stress: harms and benefits for human health. Oxid Med Cell Longev 2017; 2017: 8416763.
[http://dx.doi.org/10.1155/2017/8416763] [PMID: 28819546]

[37]   Djeridane A, Yousfi M, Brunel JM, Stocker P. Isolation and characterization of a new steroid derivative as a powerful antioxidant from *Cleome arabica* in screening the in vitro antioxidant capacity of 18 Algerian medicinal plants. Food Chem Toxicol 2010; 48(10): 2599-606.
[http://dx.doi.org/10.1016/j.fct.2010.06.028] [PMID: 20600536]

[38]   Li S, Tan J, Zeng J. XianjinWu XW, Zhang J. Antihyperglycemic and antioxidant effect of the total flavones of *Potentillakleiniana* Wight et Arn. in streptozotocin-induced diabetic rats. Pak J Pharm Sci 2017; 30(1): 171-8.
[PMID: 28603128]

[39]   Sobeh M, Mahmoud MF, Abdelfattah MAO, El-Beshbishy HA, El-Shazly AM, Wink M. Hepatoprotective and hypoglycemic effects of a tannin rich extract from *Ximenia americana* var. caffra root. Phytomedicine 2017; 33: 36-42.
[http://dx.doi.org/10.1016/j.phymed.2017.07.003] [PMID: 28887918]

[40]   Sales PM, Souza PM, Simeoni LA, Silveira D. α-Amylase inhibitors: a review of raw material and isolated compounds from plant source. J Pharm Pharm Sci 2012; 15(1): 141-83.
[http://dx.doi.org/10.18433/J35S3K] [PMID: 22365095]

[41]   Etxeberria U, de la Garza AL, Campión J, Martínez JA, Milagro FI. Antidiabetic effects of natural plant extracts via inhibition of carbohydrate hydrolysis enzymes with emphasis on pancreatic alpha amylase. Expert Opin Ther Targets 2012; 16(3): 269-97.
[http://dx.doi.org/10.1517/14728222.2012.664134] [PMID: 22360606]

[42]   Bammou M, Sellam K, El-Rhaffari L, Echchagadda G, Ibijbijen J, Nassiri L. Antibacterial activity (in vitro) of the aqueous extract of leaves of Anvillearadiata (Coss&Dur) on antibiotic-resistant bacteria. Science Lib Editions Mersenne 2014; p. 6.

[43]   Bammou M, Sellam K, El Rhaffari L, *et al.* Bioactivity of *Anvillea radiata* coss & dur. collected from the southeast of morocco. Eur Sci J 2015; 11(21): 233-44.

[44]   Elkhamass M, Oulahcen B, Lekchiri A, Sebbata A, Charhabaili Y. Stratégie de lutte contre les maladies de post-récolte des fruits d'agrumes.

[45]   Askarne L, Talibi I, Boubaker H, *et al.* Use of Moroccan medicinal plant extracts as botanical fungicide against citrus blue mould. Lett Appl Microbiol 2013; 56(1): 37-43.
[http://dx.doi.org/10.1111/lam.12012] [PMID: 23061438]

[46]   Moumou M, El Bouakher A, Allouchi H, *et al.* Synthesis and biological evaluation of 9α- and 9β-

hydroxyamino-parthenolides as novel anticancer agents. Bioorg Med Chem Lett 2014; 24(16): 4014-8.
[http://dx.doi.org/10.1016/j.bmcl.2014.06.019] [PMID: 24998377]

[47] El Bouakher A, Jismy B, Allouchi H, *et al.* Synthetic Modification of 9α- and 9β-Hydroxyparthenolide by Heck or Acylation Reactions and Evaluation of Cytotoxic Activities. Planta Med 2017; 83(7): 661-71.
[PMID: 27919107]

[48] Mishima S, Yoshida C, Akino S, Sakamoto T. Antihypertensive effects of *Brazilian propolis*: identification of caffeoylquinic acids as constituents involved in the hypotension in spontaneously hypertensive rats. Biol Pharm Bull 2005; 28(10): 1909-14.
[http://dx.doi.org/10.1248/bpb.28.1909] [PMID: 16204944]

[49] Suzuki A, Yamamoto N, Jokura H, *et al.* Chlorogenic acid attenuates hypertension and improves endothelial function in spontaneously hypertensive rats. J Hypertens 2006; 24(6): 1065-73.
[http://dx.doi.org/10.1097/01.hjh.0000226196.67052.c0] [PMID: 16685206]

[50] Agunloye OM, Oboh G, Ademiluyi AO, *et al.* Cardio-protective and antioxidant properties of caffeic acid and chlorogenic acid: Mechanistic role of angiotensin converting enzyme, cholinesterase and arginase activities in cyclosporine induced hypertensive rats. Biomed Pharmacother 2019; 109: 450-8.
[http://dx.doi.org/10.1016/j.biopha.2018.10.044] [PMID: 30399581]

[51] Kozuma K, Tsuchiya S, Kohori J, Hase T, Tokimitsu I. Antihypertensive effect of green coffee bean extract on mildly hypertensive subjects. Hypertens Res 2005; 28(9): 711-8.
[http://dx.doi.org/10.1291/hypres.28.711] [PMID: 16419643]

[52] Zhou Y, Wang S, Zhang Y. Catalytic reaction mechanism of acetylcholinesterase determined by Born-Oppenheimer ab initio QM/MM molecular dynamics simulations. J Phys Chem B 2010; 114(26): 8817-25.
[http://dx.doi.org/10.1021/jp104258d] [PMID: 20550161]

[53] Retz W, Gsell W, Münch G, Rösler M, Riederer P. Free radicals in Alzheimer's disease. J Neural Transm Suppl 1998; 54: 221-36.
[http://dx.doi.org/10.1007/978-3-7091-7508-8_22] [PMID: 9850931]

[54] Konrath EL, Passos CdosS, Klein LC Jr, Henriques AT. Alkaloids as a source of potential anticholinesterase inhibitors for the treatment of Alzheimer's disease. J Pharm Pharmacol 2013; 65(12): 1701-25.
[http://dx.doi.org/10.1111/jphp.12090] [PMID: 24236981]

[55] Pinho BR, Ferreres F, Valentão P, Andrade PB. Nature as a source of metabolites with cholinesterase-inhibitory activity: an approach to Alzheimer's disease treatment. J Pharm Pharmacol 2013; 65(12): 1681-700.
[http://dx.doi.org/10.1111/jphp.12081] [PMID: 24236980]

[56] Miyazawa M, Watanabe H, Kameoka H. Inhibition of acetylcholinesterase activity by monoterpenoids with a p-menthane skeleton. J Agric Food Chem 1997; 45(3): 677-9.
[http://dx.doi.org/10.1021/jf960398b]

[57] Seo SY, Sharma VK, Sharma N. Mushroom tyrosinase: recent prospects. J Agric Food Chem 2003; 51(10): 2837-53.
[http://dx.doi.org/10.1021/jf020826f] [PMID: 12720364]

[58] Briganti S, Camera E, Picardo M. Chemical and instrumental approaches to treat hyperpigmentation. Pigment Cell Res 2003; 16(2): 101-10.
[http://dx.doi.org/10.1034/j.1600-0749.2003.00029.x] [PMID: 12622786]

SUBJECT INDEX

A

Ability 34, 67, 68, 69, 111, 139, 150
  high glucose tolerance 111
  insulin-secretory 34
Accumulation 63, 64, 67
  lipid 64
  liver fat 64
ACE inhibitors 121
Acetylation 67
  inhibited hypertension-induced 67
Acetylcholine 149
  hydrolyzing 149
Acetylcholinesterase 149
Acid 16, 18, 21, 23, 34, 40, 44, 61, 82, 83, 89, 90, 107, 108, 127, 129, 130, 142
  Arachidic 82, 108
  ascorbic 21, 40, 129
  betulinic 82
  corosolic 34
  di-caffeoylquinic 142
  edulilic 129
  elenolic 90
  ellagic 127, 130
  gallic 127, 130
  gymnemic 16, 34
  Hexadecanoic 107
  linoleic 18, 44, 108
  maslinic 82
  myristic 108
  octadecadienoic 107
  oleanolic 83, 89, 90
  oleic 18, 44, 108
  oxoheptacosanoic 107
  oxotriaconsanoic 107
  palmitic 108
  stearic 108
  Succinic 108
  thiobarbituric 61
  ursolic 82
Acid phosphatase 66, 110
  tartrate-resistant 66
Acid-reactive substances measurement 128

Activities 43, 61, 62 65, 66, 83, 84, 86, 92, 102, 104, 106, 108, 109, 110, 111, 122, 126, 136, 145, 146, 148, 149
  anticancer 148
  anti-diabetic 104, 106, 108, 109, 111, 126
  antihyperglycemic 136
  anti-hyperglycemic 102
  anti-inflammatory 43, 83, 84, 146
  antimicrobial 84, 146
  anti-tyrosinase 136
  arginase 149
  calcium channel blockers 86, 92
  enhanced antioxidant enzymes 65
  enzymatic 61
  glucose-lowering 110, 146
  hypoglycaemic 92
  hypolipidemic 136, 145
  ligand-confining 62
  malate dehydrogenase 66
  protein tyrosine phosphatase 122
Acylation reactions 148
Adipocytes 63, 145
Adipogenesis 63, 64
  suppressed 63
Adipokines 61, 68, 69
  downregulating 69
Adiponectin secretion 63
Adipose tissue 4, 63
  dysfunction 63
  macrophages 63
Agents 6, 126
  anti-hyperlipidemic 6
  anti-inflammatory 126
Albumin 63, 106, 110
  glycated 41
Alkaline phosphatase 110
Alkaloids 7, 8, 25, 100, 102, 109, 111, 113, 119, 124, 130, 139, 150
  berberine hydrochloride 25
  harmala 124
  indole 130
  isoquinoline 7
Alzheimer's disease 150

Ameliorated macrophage infiltration 65
Anthracenosides 139
Anticholinesterase 149, 150, 151
  activity 149
  inhibitory activity 150, 151
Antidiabetic 45, 79, 89, 102, 119, 131, 145, 151
Antidiabetic 8, 44, 45, 46, 47, 126, 130
  activities 45, 46, 47, 126, 130
  agents 8
  phytomedicines 46
  phytotherapy 44
  therapy 46
Antifungal activity 125, 147
Antihypertensive 85, 86, 121, 128, 148, 149
  activity 121, 128, 148, 149
  treatment 85, 86
Antioxidants 46, 47, 68, 83, 88, 89, 92, 105, 119, 122, 127, 128, 130, 144, 145, 151
  action 68
  activity 122, 127, 128, 130, 144
  defence mechanisms 46
  enzymes 46
  properties 83
Apoptosis 88
Arteriosclerosis 120
Arthritis 102, 105, 136, 151
Autoimmunity 2
Ayurvedic medicine 15

B

Bacillus cereus 147, 150
Bacillus subtilis 146
Barberry juice (BJ) 8, 25
Bell pepper juice 7, 24
Berberis aristata extract 8, 26
Bioactive phyto-compounds 43
Bitter gourd 12, 27, 31
  consumption 27
  powder 12, 27, 31
  supplementation 27
Blood 67, 102, 110
  sugar monitoring 102
  urea nitrogen 110
  vessel morphology 67
Blood glucose 3, 7, 9, 11, 13, 14, 20, 21, 32, 43, 44, 15, 16, 21, 35, 37, 44, 70, 91, 108, 127, 128, 145
  elevated 11, 44

lower fasting 21
post prandial 7
post-prandial 13, 32, 43, 91
random 3
reduced fasting 14, 20
Blood glucose levels 7, 11, 13, 14, 18, 28, 61, 62, 89, 102, 106, 145
  changing fasting 7
  prolonged increased 102
Blood pressure 4, 7, 20, 21, 38, 43, 45, 85, 86, 87, 92, 120, 121, 128, 129, 130, 148, 149
  ambulatory 87
  arterial 148, 149
  diastolic 20, 85, 86, 87, 128, 129, 148
  homeostasis 129
  influence 38
  normalized arterial 149
  systolic 7, 85, 86, 128, 148, 149
Brewer's yeast capsule 29
Butylated hydroxyl toluene (BHT) 108, 144

C

Cancer 3, 5, 85, 86, 123, 139
  colon 123
Capsicum annuum 7, 24
Carbohydrate(s) 42, 102, 108, 122, 126, 128
  absorption, intestinal 102
  hydrolyzing enzyme 108
  intake 42, 126
  metabolism 128
  -hydrolysing enzymes inhibitors 122
Cardiac failure, preventing 70
Cardiovascular diseases 1, 3, 5, 85, 86, 92, 120, 121, 122, 123, 128
Cell death 66, 69
  apoptotic germ 66
Cell permeability, increasing 45
Cell regeneration 109, 127
  pancreatic 109
Centrifugal partition chromatography (CPC) 140
Chemical 82, 147
  composition of olive leaf 82
  fungicides 147
Chlopropamide 11
Chlorogenic acid 21, 40, 123, 142, 149
Cholesterol 15, 84, 86, 146
  plasmatic 86

factor (NF) 84
translocation 84

O

Obesity 3, 5, 12, 15, 34, 63, 120, 121, 123,
     136, 151
  high-fat diet-induced 63
Oil 23, 27, 42, 46, 79, 81, 82, 100, 139
  lemon peel 27
  volatile 139
  walnut 23, 42, 46
Oleuropein 79, 82, 83, 84, 87, 89, 91, 92
  assayed 84
  identifying 92
Oleuropein 82, 90
  aglycone 82
  effects 90
  glucoside 82
Olive leaf 84, 85, 86, 87, 90, 91, 92
  extract 85, 86, 87, 90, 91, 92
  extract supplementation 91
  phenolics 84
Olive oil 80, 81, 85, 86
Oxidation 5, 28, 41, 46, 66
  inhibiting DNA 66
  lipid 28
Oxidative stress 46, 66, 68, 89, 100, 129, 145

P

Pancreas 4, 70, 101, 102, 107, 110, 120
  damage 110
Pancreatic cells dysfunction 64
Pancreatitis 2
Penicillium italicum 147
Peroxisome 4, 61
  activating 61
  initiating 61
Phospholipase 65
Phospholipids 69
Phytochemical analysis 136, 142, 145
Phytoremedies 2, 5, 6, 43, 44, 46, 47
  plant-derived 5
  potential antidiabetic 44
Plant-based medicines 101, 102, 113
  traditional 101

Plant-derived 1, 5
  bioactive compounds 1, 5
  phytotherapy 1
Postprandial 4, 8, 15, 17, 25, 29, 35, 41, 43,
     111, 128
  blood sugar levels 111
  C-peptide 8, 25, 43
  glycemia 15
  hyperglycaemia 4
  insulin 8, 17, 25, 29, 41
Postprandial glucose 7, 14, 15, 21, 25
  decreased 15
  reduced 14
Post-prandial plasma glucose 2
Pregnancy 2, 120
Pressure 66, 86, 87, 92, 129
  diastolic 129
  intracavernosal 66
  systolic 87
Pressurized liquid extraction 141
Primary hypertension 120
Production 4, 40, 62, 63, 67, 68, 84, 110
  cytokine 62
  hepatic glucose 4, 40, 110
  prostacyclin 68
Products 85, 89, 122, 123, 125, 149
  ayurvedic 123
  natural 85, 89, 122, 125, 149
Properties 64, 81, 84, 86, 92, 119, 126
  antianxiety 119
  anti-inflammatory 64, 126
  antitumoral 84
  antiviral 119
  cholesterol-lowering 86, 92
  hypotriglyceridemic 126
Protein 22, 23
  glycation 22
  glycosylation, reduced 23
Protein kinase 46, 62, 65, 100, 102
  C (PKC) 46, 62, 65, 100, 102
Proteins 2, 9, 16, 32, 35, 41, 44, 46, 65, 68,
     82, 100, 111, 122, 126
  cAMP response element binding 65
  glycated 46
  glycated total plasma 41
  glycosylated 41
  glycosylated plasma 16, 35
  plasma 35